I Can't Walk But
I Can Crawl

Living with cerebral palsy

Joan Ross

P·C·P
Paul Chapman
Publishing

ISBN: 978-1-4129-1872-5

 Published by Lucky Duck
Paul Chapman Publishing
A SAGE Publications Company
1 Oliver's Yard
55 City Road
London EC1Y 1SP

SAGE Publications, Inc.
2455 Teller Road
Thousand Oaks, California 91320

SAGE Publications India Pvt Ltd
B-42, Panchsheel Enclave
Post Box 4109
New Delhi 110 017

www.luckyduck.co.uk

Commissioning Editor: Barbara Maines
Editorial Team: Mel Maines, Sarah Lynch, Wendy Ogden, Mike Gibbs
Designer: Helen Weller

© Joan Ross 2005
Reprinted 2007

Printed by Cromwell Press, Trowbridge, Wiltshire.

Printed on paper from sustainable resources.

Contents

Acknowledgements   vii

Foreword   ix

Cerebral Palsy, Scope and Joan by Alex White   xi

Scope's Mission   xvii

1   A New Life   1

2   School Days   9

3   See the Child, not the Disability   17

4   My New Treatment   23

5   Queen Mary's in Surrey   31

6   Little Miss Mischief   37

7   Vale Road School   45

8   Rewarding Times   53

9   Girl Guides   59

10   Rangers   65

11   Moving On   71

12   Challenge   75

13   More Education Please   81

14   My Own Brownie Pack   87

15   Bus Rides   95

16   I Want to Learn to Drive   101

17   Going on Holiday by Car   107

18   In Pursuit of a Teaching Career   113

19   Middlesex Polytechnic   119

20   Seeking Employment   127

21   A Real Job   133

22   Haringey Disability Association   141

23   Changing Cars   147

24 My Small Corner   155
25 Concern Over My Parents' Health   161
26 Problems at Home   167
27 Voluntary Work   173
28 A Break from Caring   179
29 Severance   185
30 Some Drastic Action   193
31 Vancouver and Susy from Hackney   201
Epilogue   207

This book is dedicated to my mother and my father.

Lucky Duck is more than a publishing house and training agency. George Robinson and Barbara Maines founded the company in the 1980s when they worked together as a head and as a psychologist, developing innovative strategies to support challenging students.

They have an international reputation for their work on bullying, self-esteem, emotional literacy and many other subjects of interest to the world of education.

George and Barbara have set up a regular news-spot on the website at http://www.luckyduck.co.uk/newsAndEvents/viewNewsItems and information about their training programmes can be found at www.insetdays.com

More details about Lucky Duck can be found at http://www.luckyduck.co.uk/

Visit the website for all our latest publications in our specialist topics

- Emotional Literacy
- Self-esteem
- Bullying
- Positive Behaviour Management
- Circle Time
- Anger Management
- Asperger's Syndrome
- Eating Disorders

Acknowledgements

I would like to thank the following:

The City Lit. Humanities Department Holborn.

Carol Burns, for her guidance in autobiographical writing.

John Sawyer, for keeping my computer in good running order.

Alex White at Scope, who prepared part one of my book for submission.

Vicky Keeping and Fiona McGeever at Scope.

Karol Joseph Pitra, for the lovely photographs.

Rebecca Dee, who typed for me after I stopped using Dragon Dictate.

Foreword

This book describes the life, so far, of a woman who has cerebral palsy. Her humour, strength, determination and patience shine through her testimony throughout. She is not 'brave', she simply refuses to let a condition (that many people use as an excuse for prejudice) determine her life choices. Some of the choices that she may have liked to have pursued are denied her. Yet she creates so many more choices and lives her life as fully as possible.

I had the pleasure of meeting Joan recently to discuss her book and make sure that she was happy with the edited version. When I first read the manuscript, it reminded me of being in the company of someone who was reminiscing in a very relaxed manner, maybe over a cup of tea and a slice of cake. Any attempts at changing or re-arranging this style would be so apparent, it would ruin the effect. With its relaxed style, it's an easy and absorbing read.

So why should you read this book? It's important for others to know the truth about what it has been like to be disabled in the twentieth century. By highlighting her life story, Joan's autobiography also explores attitudes, and reveals where there may still be barriers to equality. Read it if you are a non-disabled person to be motivated by an incredible woman's fight to be counted. Read it if you are disabled and have felt the unfairness of many aspects of society, to see just how the system can be beaten. Read it for the fascinating social history. Read it if you want to experience a kind of lifestyle that you may never have considered before. Read it to be inspired.

Sarah Lynch 2005

Cerebral Palsy, Scope and Joan

Cerebral palsy is not a disease or an illness. It is a physical condition that affects movement and communication. However, as Joan Ross's book proves, having cerebral palsy doesn't mean that you can't lead a full and rewarding life and achieve much more than doctors in the thirties and forties expected – and many people expect even today.

As a member of Scope and Chair of the North London Cerebral Palsy Association, Joan came to us in the hope of finding a publisher. We had just published *Can You Manage Stares?*, the autobiography of Bill Hargreaves, an amazing man with cerebral palsy who helped found the charity and whose pioneering work transformed the lives of thousands of disabled people. I had to tell Joan that Bill's book had only been published thanks to a grant from the National Lottery and that it didn't seem that publishers were interested in disabled people's lives, however remarkable.

As I write this preface to Joan's publishing debut, I'm glad that Lucky Duck has proved me wrong. Like Scope, Lucky Duck realises that stories like Joan and Bill's are important because they tell a wider public about what it is like to be disabled by society, what it is like to be written off when one is young and to struggle against other people's prejudices.

As Bill relates, in the 1950s, people with cerebral palsy like Joan were almost invisible:

The only cerebral palsied person I'd ever met in my life before was myself in the mirror, because there weren't any people with cerebral palsy in the streets. There weren't any at all. I saw one-legged men, I saw blind people, I saw people with hydrocephalus, this sort of thing, but no people with cerebral palsy. Why? Because their parents were ashamed of having their children - which was appalling.

Although things have improved and disabled people today are more visible in society, disablism – prejudice against disabled people – is rife. We at Scope define disablism as:

> … discriminatory, oppressive or abusive behaviour arising from the belief that disabled people are inferior to others.

Disablism is not a word that is recognised by the Oxford English Dictionary, but if you a disabled person you know that it exists; you encounter it every day. That's why Scope has launched the Time to Get Equal campaign to banish disablism from our society.

Once you have read Joan's book, I am sure that you will feel moved to join the campaign and help us to change people's attitudes! If you do, please go to www.timetogetequal.org.uk and lend us your support.

My conversation with Joan prompted me to approach the Heritage Lottery Fund to help Scope to uncover even more life stories of disabled people. Once we received our funding, I was very glad that Joan agreed to take part in this project, called Speaking for Ourselves, which will result in an Archive Hour radio documentary on Radio Four as well as a teaching pack for secondary schools in 2006. You can find out more via the website at www.speakingforourselves.org.uk as well as via The British Library Sound Archive (collection reference: C1134).

Joan is an ordinary person like you and I but she has faced extraordinary barriers to living a normal life. She was born in 1939 at a time of very little public awareness of the problems facing children with cerebral palsy. Parents were routinely told by doctors to have another baby and put their children with cerebral palsy in institutions.

Until the formation of Scope (then called The National Spastics Society) in 1952 and for some time after, children with cerebral palsy were regarded by the medical profession as 'ineducable'. Unusually for the time, Joan was offered a place at a local infant school. For many of her disabled peers, education in a local school, alongside friends and siblings, was a distant dream. The only school for children with cerebral palsy, St Margaret's in Croydon, could accommodate only a very limited number of children, but parents throughout the country applied for places, and a waiting list of 200 was quickly established, so great was the need.

Among the first pupils at St Margaret's were Rosemary, daughter of Ian Dawson-Shepherd, Susan, daughter of Eric Hodgson, and Alice, daughter of Alex Moira. Their parents were becoming increasingly concerned and frustrated at the lack of forward thinking, as there was no secondary education for children with cerebral palsy.

Together with the social worker, Jean Garwood, the parents met on 9 October 1951 at Eric Hodgson's isolated home at Long Lane, Croydon to discuss the creation of a grammar school for their children. This is how Scope historian Bill Elliott relates how the first meeting went:

> Their first argument centred on the proposed name for the new organisation. The chairman opted for a name with 'Spastics' in it, but the secretary and the treasurer who both disliked the word, wanted 'cerebral palsy'.
>
> The Advisor agreed because, she said, "It was the proper medical term." The argument went back and forth until Ian Dawson-Shepherd ventured that they should call themselves the National Spastics Society, which, ultimately, was agreed by all. How could they call the society National when in fact they were but a group of four people, lacking funds, sitting round a fire in a suburban house in Croydon? How could they begin their campaign without money? When no ideas were forthcoming, Ian Dawson-Shepherd, in a pseudo-dramatic gesture, pulled out a £5 note from his pocket and slapped it onto the table, saying, "There's the start." It would be nice to record that at that solemn moment they all stood up and

shook hands, their eyes shining with hope – but they didn't. Eric laughed cynically, "A fiver won't get us very far." "All right then," Ian retorted, "I'll make you a million pounds in five years." "Don't talk bloody daft, Ian," said Eric with pity.

Shortly afterwards, Ian Dawson-Shepherd wrote to the *Daily Mirror*, who agreed to publish his letter:

> A new and powerful society has been formed to press, argue and fight to get better treatment for spastic sufferers. Would you ask all sufferers or their relatives to write to the National Spastics Society at the above address and start helping the Society.

Within a few days the *Daily Mirror* had received more than 300 replies from parents, a good response for a hitherto unknown subject. The group was impressed, which was to lead later to greater co-operation with the paper. In the meantime, it gave Eric the names of 300 parents to whom he could write and suggest that they each form a local parents' group.

The inaugural meeting of the National Spastics Society was held at The Ambassadors Hotel, Southampton Row, London WC1 on 5 January 1952. From this modest start, the charity grew rapidly.

Alex White, Scope

Scope's Mission

Scope's mission is to drive the change to make our society the first where disabled people achieve full equality.

Our goals are that:

disablism is banished

all disabled people of all ages and their families enjoy their full and equal human and civil rights

all disabled people are able to exercise full personal choice and control over their own lives.

We will achieve this by:

being led by the views and lived experience of disabled people

valuing and listening to disabled families

working in alliance with disabled people and their organisations

using all our passion, professionalism, energy and resources.

In so doing we will support people with cerebral palsy, and their families, at all stages of their lives, including:

through a commitment to universal independent advocacy

by achieving excellence in our understanding and knowledge of the condition and related impairments

whilst fundamentally changing society so that people with cerebral palsy, and other conditions, can achieve their full potential and enjoy equality.

To find out more about Scope, go to
www.scope.org.uk

1
A New Life

When my nephew was born I gazed on him filled with wonder and emotion. He was the youngest child I'd ever had close contact with. What would this tiny thing, so physically perfect, be like as a person? Will he be clever and handsome? What will be his career? It was very moving to realise that in this little body was everything he'd need, given by God, to live in this world.

My sister was anxious that Andrew wouldn't be born with cerebral palsy like me. She insisted on a hospital birth for her first child. She read all about pregnancy and childbirth, wanting everything to be right.

I'm glad there were no tests during her pregnancy in 1938 that Mum could have taken to find out whether I had any physical or mental defects before I was born. I was brain damaged during birth through lack of oxygen; so my impairment wouldn't have been detected in any scan or test.

According to the Society for the Protection of Unborn Children (SPUC), there are now a growing number of tests, which aim to detect disabling conditions in unborn babies. What a terrible dilemma to have to decide whether or not to terminate a pregnancy.

Because I believe life is a very special gift from God, I am totally against abortion. Every child is a seed waiting to flourish and they all need nurturing to reach their full potential.

* * * * * * * * * *

It was 1939. I was nearly born in India. Dad had signed on for 22 years' army service and Mum had been with him in India for a few years. When war was imminent, all the women were sent back home to Britain. I was born in my Grandmother's house in Holyhead, north Wales. When Mum realised I wasn't developing at the same rate as other children my age, she suspected that I might have some kind of physical impairment.

She decided to take me to the Alder Hey children's hospital in Liverpool to try and obtain a diagnosis, and was told in no uncertain words that I would never be able to walk, that it was highly unlikely that I would grow up to recognise my parents.

Mum and I stayed in Wales until I was two. Mum's sister, Auntie Madge, had married an Englishman who was also in the army. She lived in London and suggested that Mum should take me to Great Ormond Street Children's Hospital for a second diagnosis. Once again I was diagnosed as having brain damage and they offered me treatment in the form of physiotherapy.

I lay on my back unable to sit up without support until I was nearly three. Then I learnt to crawl, and my world of childhood fantasy began. Mum and I lived with Auntie Madge until I was 12. My uncle died in a

2

prisoner of war camp. The two sisters lived together throughout the war and were, of course, a tremendous support to one another. My father was excused from service overseas. He became an army instructor in the Royal Welch Fusiliers and was stationed in Brecon, South Wales. Andrew Cruickshank and Jack Hawkins were in his regiment.

The two sisters stayed in London for most of the bombing. Great Ormond Street agreed to give me exercises and electrical massage. My mother carried me on the buses and underground twice a week to attend hospital for my treatment. She often got lost at first because she didn't know her way around London; this caused a lot of amusement between the two sisters. Mum, however, enjoyed sightseeing in the City. We were often out all day.

I loved living with Auntie Madge. I had a friend called Margaret living close by. Saturday afternoons were usually boring if I had no one to play with. One particular Saturday my boredom was ended when suddenly the doorbell rang shrilly. A voice shouted, 'Are Redskin Joan Ross and Redskin Margaret Jones at home?' Auntie Madge stood dumbfounded when she opened the front door to a man dressed as a Native American. 'I am Big Chief I-Spy! They've both won a competition.'

Auntie Madge often told this story. 'You could have knocked me down with a feather from his headdress!' she would say. Margaret and I had joined the I-Spy Club in the *Daily Telegraph*. I was eight, Margaret nine.

Auntie Madge rushed down the road to fetch Margaret who was washing her hair. She arrived at my home flushed with excitement, with a towel round her head.

This is all I can remember about Big I-Spy's visit. I have no idea what the competition was about, or which prizes Margaret and I won. Auntie Madge had encouraged us to join the club. We loved the I-Spy books: *I-Spy at the Seaside*, *I-Spy in the City*. There were secret codes to crack.

Auntie Madge first worked in a factory making electrical goods. Then she passed her civil service exam for the Ministry of Agriculture and Fisheries. I loved to watch her get ready for work, putting on make-up and stroking her eyebrows with her wet fingers. Her silk petticoat shimmered as she moved. I decided that when I grew up I would work in the civil service. I would crawl to the bus stop, climb onto the bus, and work in the same ministry as my Auntie, counting chickens, eggs, and cows. I would wear make-up. It never occurred to me on rainy days that I would get splashed while I knelt at the bus stop. I would not be able to wear the smart costumes and nylon stockings worn by Auntie Madge.

My mother and Auntie Madge were very different in looks and personality. Auntie was very fastidious about her clothes and went to the hairdresser's regularly. Mum was very easy-going about everything. My aunt was a worrier; it annoyed her that my mother was so laid-back. My mother's chief concern was my welfare, health and treatment. My auntie wanted to organise my mother. She would have a go at her for not writing

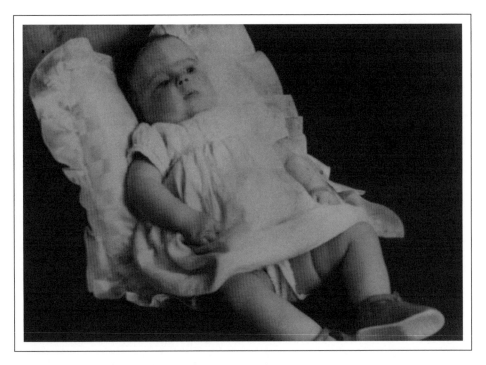

Me, nine months old, 1939.

regularly to my grandparents in Wales. 'What's the use of me writing to them, when you tell them my business anyway?' Mum retorted.

My mother and Auntie Madge were very brave staying in London throughout the Second World War. They had no relations in London, only Uncle Alan's parents. Auntie Madge had to do 'fire watch duty' throughout the war. At the beginning of the war, we always went to the cellar as soon as the air raids started. One night, when the siren went off, Mum panicked. She pushed my aunt flying to the ground, grabbed hold of me and rushed down to the cellar. Apparently, my aunt was only wearing her vest at the time. I remember Auntie Madge repeatedly reminding my mother of this incident, which was always accompanied by hysterical laughter from them both.

As the war went on, we stopped going down to the cellar. I lay in bed listening to bombs falling in the distance. It was just part of my life. I wasn't really frightened because I had grown so used to it. I was upset when Wilson's, a large retail store in Crouch End Broadway, was hit by a bomb and completely destroyed by fire. Mum, Auntie Madge and I gazed down onto the shopping centre from my bedroom window. We had a good view because we lived on a hill. The whole sky seemed to be lit up from the flames. I thought about all the lovely dolls in Wilson's and it broke my heart at the thought of them being burnt. Mum took me the next day to see what had happened to the dolls. She tried to reassure me that the kind firemen had rescued them.

The Toy Shop

Mum, Mum, look, look, the dolls! The dolls!
Hush child, they'll be all right,
They'll be safe; the fireman will save them.
I look down from my bedroom window.
Below, the sky is red with flames.
Tears pour down my cheeks.
How will I sleep tonight?
Mum, Mum, take me in the morning
To see if the dolls are all right.
We went. All was bare, and black.

(Wilson's Retail Store was bombed and destroyed in February 1944)

My mother hated her Welsh name, Blodwen. She was embarrassed about giving her name to English people. They would ask her to spell it and this made her even more embarrassed so she gave herself a French name, 'Blanche'. The trouble was she didn't always tell my aunt what she had done. One day, when my Auntie Madge was at the hairdresser's, the hairdresser asked, 'How did Blanche like her hairdo?' My aunt looked puzzled and did not answer. 'Your sister, Blanche,' the hairdresser said.

2
School Days

In 1945, education was not compulsory for disabled children. Mum rebuffed this with some disdain. She was determined that I should go to school. When I was one she took me to the Alder Hey Children's Hospital, Liverpool, and was told by the children's specialist that I was mentally retarded and would never be able to recognise my parents.

Mum must have become aware of some degree of intelligence during my second year. Dad had signed up for 22 years in the army so Mum had to fight my battles alone. My Welsh grandmother recommended that I should be introduced to the Christian faith and start going to Sunday School. Mum thought this would teach me to mix with other children. I started at the age of three. I was taken in my large pram, accompanied by Margaret, who was a year older than me and lived on the same road. She was my close childhood friend and played a large part in my early education.

The Sunday School class was held in the vicarage. I remember the teacher well: she had very round spectacles and rosy cheeks. I loved singing the hymns. 'Jesus Bids Us Shine' was one of my favourites with the line, 'You in your small corner and I in mine'. I felt sure it referred to the corner in the living room at home where I played with my toys.

Mum thought that I had a better chance of an education in a private school so she started saving towards this when I was very young. It must have been very difficult with her small army pension. However, the private school close to where we lived refused to take me.

Undaunted, Mum set off to the Education Office. 'That Ross woman is here again,' she heard someone say. 'Yes, and I will be here again tomorrow and the next day, until you offer a place for my daughter at school,' Mum insisted.

Mum had found a local infant school with buildings all on one level. The head teacher had agreed to accept me on the condition that Mum provided welfare and personal care throughout the day. I was put in a class taught by one of the older teachers. Mum was promised that they would teach me to read. Dad made a tray to tie on my chair to use as a desk. My large pushchair was called 'The Spitfire' after the British fighter plane used in the Second World War.

All went well for six weeks. Then, I announced that I had left school. I would not say why. Eventually, my mum found out what was wrong. 'They call me 'baby' because I am in a pushchair,' I said. Mum went to speak to the head teacher. She told my mum that if she could persuade me to come back to school, she would sort it out. I don't know how Mum managed to persuade me to return to school. The day I returned, the headmistress explained in assembly that there was one little girl who was in a pushchair because her legs did not work properly and she was unable to walk. She said that I was very clever and certainly not a baby. After this I loved school, especially the stories.

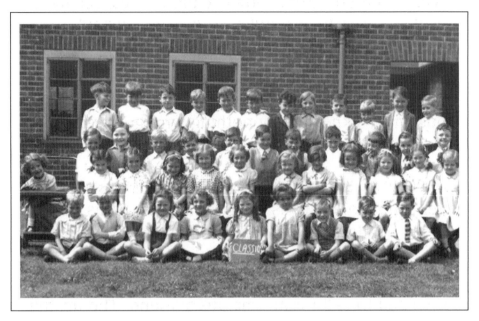

Me with my class at the local infant school, 1946.

My first teacher, Mrs Oakley, was rather fat with her hair brushed back from her face and tied in a small bun at the back. At playtime, two girls from my class were chosen to push me round the back of the school where each classroom had a small garden. I enjoyed this very much. The two girls I remember best were Gwen and Pat. At lunchtime, after feeding me my lunch, Mum took me into the playground. She walked me round the playground supporting me under the arms. I loved joining in the singing games: 'The big ship sails through the alley, alley-o' and 'Poor Jenny is a-weeping'. I was so absorbed in these singing games that I forgot I was being held by Mum, and was completely oblivious of my disability.

Inevitably, there were times when I was aware that I was different from other children, especially on meeting a new friend. 'Why can't you walk? Why can't you talk properly?' I was constantly being asked. 'I can't walk, but I can crawl,' I answered. I had special trousers made with padded knees after once getting housemaid's knee. I saw nothing wrong in walking on my knees. They seemed just as good as feet to me.

I often heard my friends arranging to call for each other after school and this is something I felt I was missing out on. I had two friends who came to my home to play with me and I also was taken to their homes to play, but I could not go and call for them. To compensate, I often pretended to call for an imaginary friend. The upstairs maisonette where I lived had large rooms with large fireplaces and a bell at the side. I imagined that this was a front door of a friend's house. This was a game that I played on days when I had nobody to play with.

One day, in desperation, I said to my mum, 'I want to go and call for my friend Margaret on my own.' To my surprise, my mum picked me up and carried me downstairs and set me down on the pavement. Delighted, I crawled towards Margaret's house. I had not gone very far when a workman stopped me. 'You naughty girl, crawling in the street – look at your shoes! Get up and walk.' We glared at each other. Then I crawled onwards to Margaret's house. I arrived at the gate and climbed up the first large step, and on to the next step. Hooray! I was outside the front door. Then I had a great disappointment. I could not reach the doorbell.

There was no alternative but to bang on the door with my fist. I seemed to bang on the door for ages. Then at last Margaret's mother opened the door. 'Oh it's you Joan, I thought it was a dog.' I was disgusted with her and I suppose this was one of the first occasions that I felt different from other children. Margaret was out.

I looked forward to Dad coming home on leave. Entertainment was high on the agenda. We always went either to Finsbury Park Empire or Wood Green Empire. At home the wireless was our chief form of entertainment. I loved the variety shows. The comedians always made me laugh. I also loved all kinds of music on the wireless, especially Joe Loss and his jazz band. I used to jig to the music on my knees. My favourite comedians were Nat Mills and Bobby, Charlie Chester, Norman Evans, Arthur Askey, Jimmy Jewel and Ben Wallace. I also enjoyed listening to the ventriloquist act, 'Educating Archie' with Peter Brough and Archie Andrews.

To see all the people on stage in a live performance was wonderful. When I was very young Dad always asked me as soon as he came home, 'Want to see girls dancing?' I nodded, 'Yes,' excitedly. Wood Green Empire was a 45-minute walk. I was taken there in my pushchair. Finsbury Park Empire was further away, so Dad carried me on the bus.

As I grew older, a definite favourite was Nat Mills and Bobby, a slapstick act. Either they made a cake or decorated a room. There was flour or wallpaper paste all over the place and on themselves. I laughed out very loud. Nat Mills and Bobby were famous for saying, 'Let's get on with it.' I knew their act by heart. I acted their performance word for word for Mum and Dad when I got home, encouraged by their shrieks of laughter, especially Mum's. However, I was a little sorry I couldn't clap my hands after each act, or stand up for 'God Save the Queen' at the end of the show. I tried banging the back of my right hand with the palm of my left hand but it didn't make much of a clap.

When Dad was home for more than a weekend, he met me from school and took me to the park. I went on the swings, the ones with bars so I wouldn't fall off. I enjoyed going on the slide and on the roundabout. Dad was a terrible tease and made me cross, especially when he threatened to go home, leaving me in the park. He never went out of sight so I wasn't too worried. Of course I told my um what he did when I got home and enjoyed seeing him being told off. Brother to four sisters, it was not surprising that Dad was such a tease. 'Your Dad was such a naughty boy when he was young – once he lit a fire in his mother's cupboard,' Mum used to say to shame him.

Dad was only average in height. His best feature was his brown wavy hair. I loved playing hairdressers, brushing or combing his hair, which must have been very painful for him due to my clumsy hands. He had pale blue eyes and a dimple in the middle of his chin. He was a little vain and would stand in front of the mirror, pushing his hair into the waves, using a little water and brilliantine. If Mum caught him, she chuckled mockingly. Dad wasn't much of a talker, more of a listener. Some people had the impression Dad was not very sociable.

I loved Dad telling me stories that he made up. They were about a little girl called Mary, who he knew in the army. I was jealous of Mary. Why did Dad know so much about Mary? Why didn't he ever bring her home? Why didn't I meet her, when I visited Dad where he was stationed in south Wales? Nevertheless, I enjoyed hearing about Mary's adventures. They were quite scary. She was always getting lost or falling down a hole and getting stuck, or climbing too high up a tree and having to be rescued.

3
See the Child, not the Disability

My birthday is a week before Christmas so I always had a party. Margaret and her brother Peter came. Also Tommy from across the road. He always invited me to his bonfire night party. Some children came from my class at school. Pat and her sister Christine, who I played with in Holyhead, were also invited. Lorna, another friend, came too. She was a year younger than me and played with me sometimes. As soon as Lorna came into the room she went on her knees and crawled everywhere, just like me.

Party food wasn't very exciting during the 1940s. Food was still rationed until 1954. I remember how excited everyone was the first time bananas were in the shops and, when the first ice-cream parlour opened, Margaret and I went there for ice cream and a coke.

We didn't have a fridge. In the cold month of December Mum managed to make a jelly and blancmange. They set all right in the cold cellar. Auntie Madge made some sponge butterfly cakes with butter cream inside. There were fish paste sandwiches and syrup ones.

I didn't like food very much. I couldn't swallow solid food until I turned five. I lived on milky food, such as rice puddings, egg custard and Robinson's Groats. The best thing about parties was the games. 'Squeak Piggy Squeak' and 'Pass the Parcel' were my favourites.

When we were older, Margaret and I planned the games for my birthday party. Our favourite was 'Murder in the Dark'. We also liked making up forfeits. Margaret took me shopping for the party. We bought coloured paper to make paper chains for decorations. One day, it started raining when we were coming home. One of our neighbours stopped his car to offer us a lift. Margaret refused; she had been warned never to accept a lift. Margaret ran home as fast as her little legs could carry her, pushing me in my 'Spitfire'. Mum said it would have been all right to accept a lift because we knew the driver.

I loved going out with Margaret on Saturdays. Auntie Madge started giving us sixpence a week pocket money. One November we were coming home when an old man said to Margaret, 'Want a penny for the guy?' Margaret was furious and gave him a right telling off. 'Hey, Mister, you ought not to make fun of my friend just because her legs don't work properly and she can't walk.' I am sure he'd only meant to make me laugh, and he succeeded. I giggled all the way home, which seemed to make Margaret even more cross.

There was one neighbour who didn't make me laugh. Every time I met her she said, 'I'll give you sixpence when you get out of that chair and run up this road.' I was

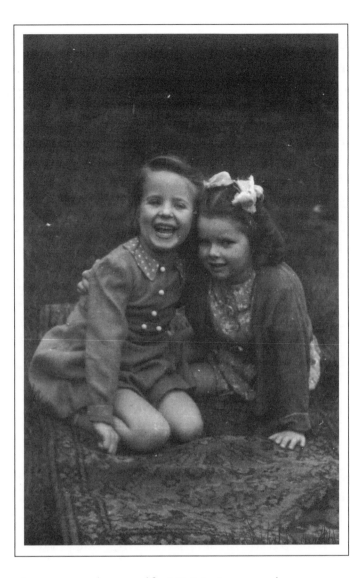

Lorna and myself, 1944. Lorna always
stayed on her knees to play with me.

disgusted with her. 'Silly woman,' I thought to myself.
'She can keep her sixpence.' Mum always took a lot
of trouble to dress me in pretty clothes. She wanted
people to see the child, not the disability. It upset her
to see a disabled child whose parents hadn't bothered

to dress her or him nicely. She had all the natural pride of a parent.

I often got into trouble for not answering people when they spoke to me. Mum wanted people to know I was intelligent. If I sat with my mouth wide open, she said, 'Stop catching flies.' People thought this sounded cruel. I appreciated her eagerness to make me aware of my appearance and the good impression this had on other people.

When I was very young, Mum found that my eyes weren't focusing properly. I was looking at everything with my chin tucked in my chest and my eyes raised upwards. She tied a scarf with a very big knot under my chin, forcing it up. It must have been during the winter! This is how I learnt to focus my eyes properly.

The advantage of being able to crawl around my home, rather than sitting in a wheelchair all day, was being able to get into mischief. Once, I washed some dolls' clothes in the water Mum had left while she was hanging out washing. I hid them. They were found some time later in a maggoty state and were destroyed. When I was staying with my granny I hid her cat in the cupboard where I knew she'd once had her kittens because I wanted her to have some more!

I appreciated just how much freedom I'd had as a child when I met Gwen in my late teens. Gwen was about 15 years older than me. Her mother had died when she was a baby. Her father remarried when she was two years old. I think that being deaf must have been a great handicap. She wore a hearing aid. She was intelligent and sensitive. Gwen was short in stature. Neatly dressed, she had a petite figure. She had brown wavy hair with a fringe. She wore glasses and had a mature expressive face. Her mobility seemed good enough to be able to get out and about on her own. She lived on a main road with many different bus routes.

I was amazed to learn how much Gwen's parents dominated this young woman. She had never voted in an election. She lacked confidence both intellectually and physically. She never went out for a walk on her own. I found this so frustrating at a time when I was exploring my own capabilities. I wanted Gwen to do the same things as me. I tried hard to persuade her to become more independent. I realized the impossibility of this task when I was invited to tea with Gwen and her parents. They seemed to be watching every move she made. At the tea table Gwen jumped every time she dropped a crumb. Her parents' manner did much to explain why Gwen was so jumpy and nervous. I suspect I was considered a bad influence on their daughter, always putting ideas into her head about becoming more independent. Sadly, Gwen eventually had several nervous breakdowns. A friend took me in her 'bubble car' to visit her while she was being treated for one of them. It was very sad to see her in a mental hospital, obviously heavily sedated. I often wonder whether her life would have been different if her real mother hadn't died when she was young.

4
My New Treatment

One day my consultant asked to see my mother. He told her about an article that had just been published in *The Lancet*. It was about a new treatment for my condition. He recommended that I should be referred for this treatment. My mother was all for this.

A few weeks later, the consultant told my mother that there was a very long waiting list for the consultation. Also, the treatment was undertaken in a hospital owned by London County Council: Queen Mary's Hospital in Surrey. Middlesex County Council administered where we lived. I was now five and had started school. My mother stopped taking me to Great Ormond Street Hospital because I had not made much progress. Now she felt for the first time ever that this new treatment was definitely for me. She was determined to enable me to receive it. To achieve this was no mean feat. My parents decided to seek help from our Member of Parliament.

I have heard this story related by my mother to people many times, with such pride: 'Cyril wore his uniform, being a regular soldier, when we visited our MP. I'm sure it helped.' I also went along with my parents to see David Gammons. He must have been impressed with me because Mum said he promised, 'to raise the matter in the House of Commons, if necessary'.

At last, I received a private consultation with Mrs Eirene Collis, who had developed the new treatment, after studying under Dr Winthrop M. Phelps in America during the Second World War.

There were times when my mother wanted me to speak clearly, and other times when she wished I hadn't spoken quite so clearly. Once, after arriving home from the shops, she sat me down at the bottom of the stairs, as usual, intending to take the shopping up first. Instead, she paused to listen to a brother and sister talking. They lived in the flat below us. I got tired of waiting, so I said, 'You go upstairs, Mum, and I'll listen to these people for you.' I never saw Mum run up the stairs so quickly.

I also embarrassed Mum during my examination with Mrs Collis. I told her that marks on my body were due to flea bites from the cat. After hearing this, Mrs Collis didn't want to see my school reports. She said, 'There are no questions about this child's intelligence.' She thought I would respond well to treatment. I was offered treatment as an outpatient, at the age of nine, under very unusual conditions. My mother was advised that, since my Dad was in the army, and there were no other children, and we didn't have our own home for Mum to worry about, we should take up lodgings near the hospital. Also, Mum should work voluntarily at the special unit (as it was known), learning all she could about my treatment. My disability had a new name:

cerebral palsy. Up to now, I had mostly been referred to as having infantile paralysis. Apparently, there are five types of cerebral palsy, each having its own terminology according to which part of the brain is damaged. My type is called athetoid because the brain damage is at the base of the skull and controls my muscles.

Before starting treatment, we spent a day looking around the cerebral palsy unit. I had such good feelings about the place. I felt this was a place of achievement.

Mum found lodgings near to the hospital with an elderly lady in a quiet residential street close to the hospital. She had a shock when she found the children on the unit didn't all come from London. They were from all parts of the British Isles. Andrew and his mother were from Warrington, Dorothy and her mother from Belfast, Michael and his mother from County Durham, John and his mother from Gateshead. Like me, they had all been selected for treatment.

Mrs Collis was not a qualified doctor, but only a therapist. Therefore she lacked status with the medical profession and could not get the staff she required to carry out her treatment. Ideally, she wanted at least one member of staff for every two children. Her solution was to recruit mothers to work voluntarily on her unit. The unit was not set up as a hospital ward because the children were not sick. There was no staff in nurses' uniforms, only orderlies in green overalls and physiotherapists, mostly Norwegian, who wore white coats. She also had a speech therapist, secretary and carpenter. The carpenter's job was to make chairs and

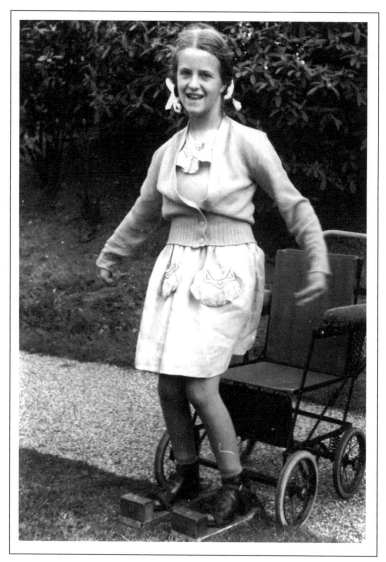

Standing alone for the first time, 1950.

tables to the exact measurements of each child. He also
made special equipment, such as trays with holes for
a plate and mug to keep them still, and cutlery with
thick handles. He also made 'skis' for children who
couldn't put their heels on the floor. These were made

from special wooden planks, joined by a steel bar, with weights behind our heels and wooden blocks with holes to place wooden poles. These were made to our correct height with straps we could put our hands through to hold the poles. We were taught to stand up holding the poles in front of a full-length mirror. This is how I eventually learnt to walk. The method of treatment was very similar to what is known today as Conductive Education, using the intelligent part of the brain to correct inappropriate movements and the positions of limbs. Therefore, Mrs Collis was very selective about choosing her patients, preferring the most intelligent. She was against any corrective surgery, splints or callipers. Mirrors were very important in the treatment room, making us aware of incorrect positions.

When I first started at the cerebral palsy unit in Queen Mary's Hospital, my disability was quite considerable. I couldn't sit or stand unsupported. I dribbled profusely. At first, I was stopped from using pencils and pens because they caused me extreme muscle tension and made me dribble. I stopped dribbling after only six weeks in the unit. I had to learn to do everything all over again, in a relaxed way. This needed much concentration at first, while it formed a pattern in the intelligent part of my brain. Then, with time, each process became automatic. Mum was very strict with me. She constantly reminded me to relax, swallow my saliva, and do things the correct way. It made her very angry when she caught me dribbling. 'Don't tell me I'm wasting two years in Carshalton for nothing,' she often said. Mum was very enthusiastic about my new treatment. She attended many of Mrs Collis's lectures. She constantly explained my treatment to everybody, whether they were interested or not! I naturally absorbed this information and put it to good use throughout my life.

Wearing skis and sitting on a chair specially made for me greatly improved my balance. To allow the physiotherapist to see my muscles working, I had to be completely naked for my physiotherapy. This took me a while to get used to. Learning to relax and breathe deeply was hard work at first. I learnt to fall from a sitting position onto the floor, which prepared me for falls when I learnt to stand and walk. I was also taught to sit cross-legged, like a tailor, which helped me to sit on the ground unsupported. It did much to strengthen the muscles in my back. After about a year, during my physiotherapy, my skis were taken off. I had to try to keep my heels flat on the floor without them. After a short while, I managed it. In my second year in the cerebral palsy unit, I started to learn to stand. Using the poles in my skis, I was helped to stand up in front of a mirror. My physiotherapist then worked on me like an artist, to attain perfection. It took immense concentration on my part. Any distraction, like the slightest noise or anyone coming into the treatment room caused me to fall over. My physiotherapist touched my knees, reminding me to straighten my legs. She moved my arms, stuck out like a penguin, to my sides. I wanted to leave my arms sticking out because it helped my balance. It was almost impossible to keep them down by my sides. Perspiration poured from my forehead.

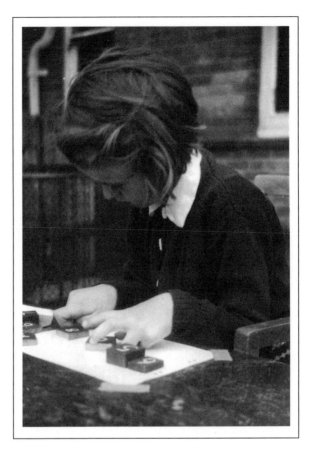

At school, 1949. Using bricks
for arithmatic because I am not
allowed to use a pencil.

5
Queen Mary's in Surrey

I thought Queen Mary's Hospital was so large, almost a village but without shops or a pub. Its entrance was up a long drive past the gatehouse. On our first morning early in January 1948, everywhere was white with frost and very cold. Nurses rushed past wearing thick heavy cloaks.

The wards were single-storey buildings set in unnamed streets, named alphabetically and by number. The cerebral palsy unit was known as C8. There was a school, a chapel, a meeting hall and a dental surgery, which, once visited, all the children hated. The cerebral palsy unit had one classroom for about ten children aged from five to ten years old. We had two teachers. I was the only child in my class who, having attended school since the age of five, read fluently. Mum was very proud of this.

Our lessons consisted of arithmetic, art, nature study, music and reading. We also had stories read to us. Most children were not allowed to use pencils, pens or paint brushes because our tight grip on them caused too much muscle tension. The basis of our treatment was learning to relax. In our arithmetic lesson, large sheets of paper with sums written on them were taped on to

31

the desk. We used small bricks with numbers painted on them to put in our answers. In our art lesson, we did finger painting using powder paints in baking trays. We dipped our fingers in the paints and painted on large sheets of paper that were taped on to the desk. We also worked with clay, which was a very good way of learning to use both hands. I mostly made ashtrays and small pots.

My closest friend was Dorothy from Belfast. Our mothers became good friends too. Eventually we shared a flat together in Wallington and travelled by train to and from Carshalton, which was great fun. Dorothy and I loved living together. We were just like sisters.

While in Queen Mary's I developed an interest in classical music. My favourite composer was Handel, influenced by listening to his Water Music played on bamboo pipes by children lying on their beds at a music festival in the hospital. It was a very moving experience, even to a ten year old, hearing these children produce such beautiful sounds from their sickbeds. I learnt all about Handel's life and how his Water Music had been written for King George II, who commissioned him to write this music for a royal boat trip down the River Thames.

My worst experience in Queen Mary's was my first visit to the dentist. Dorothy and I went together, accompanied by Mum. We were both due to have some teeth out while under sleeping gas. Dorothy was very upset. She had been to the dentist before. The sister in charge was a real ogre. She put large plastic bibs on both of us, which made Dorothy scream even more. 'Do you have to put the bib on the girls so soon?' my mother asked, 'They must get used to it,' replied the arrogant sister. I hated the gas and I struggled against it. It seemed like ages before I fell unconscious. I hated the smell of rubber. Afterwards I always hated the smell of my hot water bottle.

On our way back to the unit from school for our lunch we had to pass the dentist, which tormented us. If we caught sight of the sister near the window we trembled with fear. Her dyed blonde hair and distinct nurse's uniform made her very easy to recognize even through frosted glass. Our mothers always pushed us side by side so we could talk to one another.

During my stay in Queen Mary's the children in the cerebral palsy unit were given money for some days out. We went to Hayling Island, which had a beautiful sandy beach. Mum and I were amused and full of admiration watching my friend Andrew using a bucket and spade with his feet. I have since learnt that, when your hands don't work, feet make a very good substitute.

One of the children on the unit came from a farming family. We were invited to spend a day on the farm. We had a lovely lunch in a typical farm kitchen and were shown all the farm animals. Once a year, a fair came to the hospital. All the children who were in-patients had new clothes for the occasion. They all looked very pretty. The little girls wore gingham dresses in different colours. The little boys wore matching cotton shorts and checked shirts. The fair had everything from swinging boats to a merry-go-round and coconut shies.

Mum and I often went to London for the weekend to see Auntie Madge. This involved a train journey to London Bridge, then the Underground to Highgate. Now I had a wheelchair, having out-grown my Spitfire. Dorothy and her mother sometimes came, too. There was no such thing as access for disabled people on public transport. However, fellow passengers got used to seeing us as regular travellers on Friday nights and Monday mornings. One or two people looked out for us and helped carry me up the steps and escalators in my wheelchair. Some people gave me money for ice-cream or sweets. In those days, it wasn't considered patronising to do this.

Dorothy's mum became quite ill while we were sharing the same flat in Wallington, so Mum looked after Dorothy for a while. Once Mum took Dorothy and me, single-handedly, in two wheelchairs, to London for the weekend. Auntie Madge had a new boyfriend who was Polish and called Karol. Karol met us at Highgate Tube Station. I have never heard of anyone taking two children in wheelchairs on the Tube, single-handedly, but the mothers on the cerebral palsy unit were quite adept at pushing two wheelchairs at once.

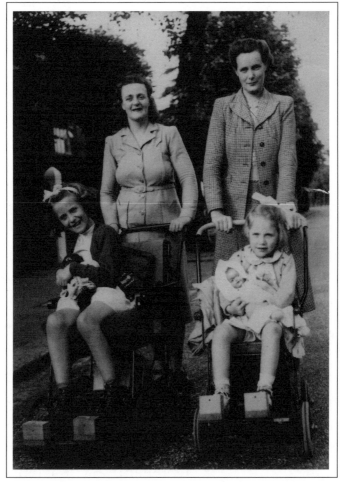

Dorothy and her mother with myself and my mother.

6
Little Miss Mischief

In 1951, when I was eleven, Mum found that she was pregnant, expecting a baby in December. There was much concern in the family. Grandmother asked, 'How will Blod cope with two children?' My Granddad was afraid I would be neglected. My mother was worried she might have another disabled child. It was thought that my disability was caused because I had weighed nine pounds and my mother has a small pelvis. My brain was damaged through lack of oxygen at birth.

My excitement at receiving this wonderful news was overshadowed by being told I would be away from home for eight weeks. There were many other problems around my mum's pregnancy. Each day she continued to carry me up and down two flights of stairs. I had just started a new school for disabled children. On the seventh month of the pregnancy someone from the Education Department came twice a day on school days to carry me to and from the coach. Auntie Madge wanted to marry again and felt it was time we had our own home. So Mum and Dad applied for a ground floor council flat. The application for this required a few doctors' certificates, so that we could be re-housed on medical grounds.

Naturally, Mum needed much reassuring that the baby would be born normally. She was promised the best medical attention at the birth. Her hospital consultant recommended that my mother should be admitted into hospital one month before the baby was born and she would stay in hospital for one month afterwards. Mum's age was also against her. She was 38.

None of my family offered to look after me while Mum was in hospital so I had to leave home for the first time. It was probably the saddest time of my life. I was sent to The Stamford Hill Cripple Home in Thorpe Bay, Essex. This was a large house on the seafront. There was a wishing well in the front garden for people to throw money in. The sign 'John Groom's Cripple Home' was written on a large board over the front door. A matron who always wore a white coat like a doctor ran it.

All the rooms were decorated in brown paint and faded floral wallpaper. The dining room served as a playroom during the day. I brought my own games to play with. The playroom was bare. We listened to Children's Hour on the wireless while we ate our tea. I was there for my twelfth birthday and at Christmas there was no special party for me, no presents or Christmas dinner. There were no Christmas decorations or even a Christmas tree and no extra presents other than those from my family. Most of the children, about 12 in all, had come from a boarding school. Presumably they had no homes to go to. Most were very disabled. I remember that we were taken to a musical called Mr Cinders. A song from that show, which summed up my mood was, 'Even though

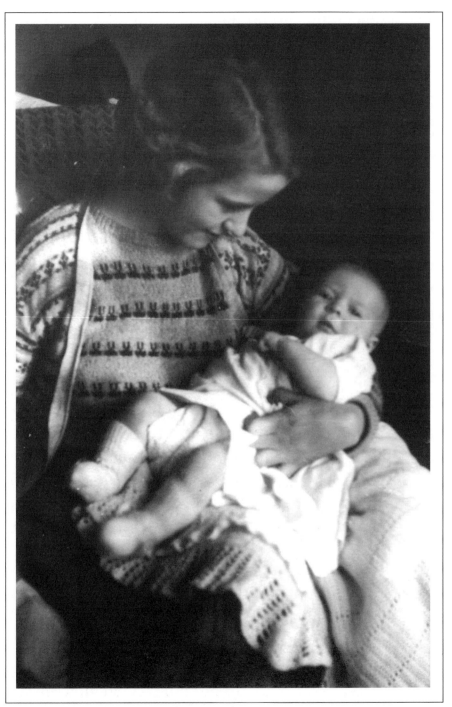

Me and baby Margaret, 1952. I wanted a photo holding my new sister just like Princess Elizabeth holding Prince Charles.

the darkest clouds are in the sky, you mustn't sigh, and you mustn't cry – spread a little happiness and you'll get by.'

Four days after Christmas I was told I had a new baby sister. I was taken out to buy her a card and a present of baby talcum powder in a pink plastic teddy. That was a happy day.

At first I cried every day. I was not used to staying in my wheelchair all day when I was not in school. I was not allowed to crawl to the places I wanted to go to indoors. I was not taken to the toilet when I needed to and, consequently, I often wet myself and got told off. In the afternoons there was only one elderly person on duty who refused to take me to the toilet. The food was very sparse and I went to bed hungry. The last meal was at 5 pm. It consisted of bread and jam. I hated to be washed and dressed by the other people. I felt I was being washed with a dry flannel.

The best day of the week was when Auntie Madge visited me on Saturdays. We went to Southend-on-Sea and had a fish and chip lunch followed by cream doughnuts. When Auntie Madge visited my mother she pretended that I was very happy where I was staying because she didn't want to upset her.

I returned home when my baby sister, Margaret, was a month old. I longed to hold her but every time I held her she screamed. 'My sister doesn't like me,' I grizzled. I wanted a photograph taken, holding her draped in a shawl, just like Princess Elizabeth holding

Prince Charles. When the baby finally got used to my 'spastic grip' and felt safe on my lap, Margaret stopped crying. We had our photograph taken just the way I had wished. My sister was very fair and had rosy cheeks. Mum said the nurses always wanted to borrow her to show their mothers how to bath new babies.

In 1952 we moved into our new council flat. Margaret was only one month old. Dad had three more years in the army, so Mum had to manage single-handed. The council offered no home help to look after Margaret and me. Money was very short. Mum only had her army allowance to live on, which was about £12 a week. Our council rent of two pounds, six shillings and eight pence took some finding every week.

Our flat had two large bedrooms and a large living room-cum-dining room. All the walls were painted white, a welcome contrast to the drab interior colours of the war years. We had two large balconies, one led from the kitchen and the other could be entered from the living room or the main bedroom. Both balconies had window boxes. We were the first tenants to move into this new block of 24 flats built to replace a row of houses that had been demolished by a bomb in the war. It was set back from the main road, situated in beautifully landscaped gardens with lawns, shrubs and rose bushes.

The King died on 5 February 1952. For what seemed like a long period the music on the wireless was very morbid. We didn't have a television. Everything stopped for the mourning of the dead King. February was a very cold month with heavy snowfalls and ice. Our heating was provided by an Ideal coke boiler in the kitchen that also heated our water. It was very temperamental and difficult to light and keep burning, depending on the direction of the wind and the quality of coke. Eventually Dad bought an oil stove that Mum often carried, lit, from room to room. We had a coal fire in the living room. We didn't have a washing machine. Mum boiled clothes in a bucket on the gas stove. Eventually she bought a gas boiler for washing our clothes, which turned the kitchen into a Turkish bath. There were very strict rules for tenants. Each tenant was allocated one day a week to hang washing out on the drying ground. Auntie Madge dried much of the baby's washing around her coal fire in the evenings.

On Sundays, when Margaret was a few months old, she was able to sit on my lap in my wheelchair. We visited Auntie Madge and stayed for our lunch and tea. She brought a television in time for the Coronation and it was strange watching children's television when I was used to listening to Children's Hour on the wireless.

I had to have some dental treatment soon after Margaret was born. After my bad experience of dentists in the cerebral palsy unit I didn't trust the school dentist. I liked the local dentist who took some teeth out by gas. It was much better than my first experience. Unfortunately, Mum had to leave the baby indoors alone when she took me to the dentist as she couldn't manage to take us both. A neighbour told Mum she had heard the baby crying. Mum never left my sister at home alone again.

Soon we had our own television and we stopped going out on Sundays. I started attending a Sunday school at a mission hall near home. The people there were very kind. During the summer one lady organised a group of people to push me to Hampstead Heath for a picnic when she realised my mother couldn't take me out very much.

Margaret was a very advanced baby. She never crawled. She just moved backwards on her tummy. She often got herself stuck under furniture. When she was seven months old she began to practise standing in her cot. Two months later, she was walking everywhere. Mum marvelled at her development. When Margaret started to walk she was mischievous and into everything. I had a chair in the bathroom. She pulled it towards the washbasin and stood on it to play with water. Mum used to ask me where the baby was, and a little voice would pipe up, 'Leave her!' We guessed she was up to mischief. Whenever I told Mum about something the baby was doing wrong she would say, 'Oh, leave her.'

I suppose I was like a second mother to Margaret when she was very young, teaching her all sorts of things and correcting bad behaviour. She was a very lively, healthy little girl. She loved it when Mum raised her voice at me. Running into the room, she'd say, 'What's Joan done wrong? Isn't she a naughty girl?'

I appreciated her more as the years went by. She was a great companion and ally. Nobody should be an only child, especially if they are disabled. She has enriched my life in so many ways.

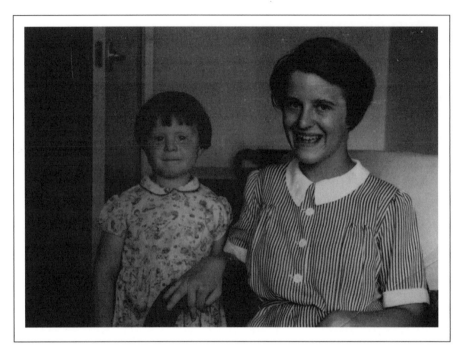

My little sister loved it when Mum raised her voice at me.

7
Vale Road School

After leaving the cerebral palsy unit, I spent a few months at home before I started the Vale Road School for Physically Handicapped Children. I was eleven. I was collected from home every morning just after 8 a.m. and arrived home again at about 4.30 p.m. The coach belonged to a private company. These coaches did day trips to the seaside in the summer. Most of the other children travelled to school from different boroughs in grey coaches belonging to the council.

Vale Road School had been converted from a Victorian building and used as a fire station during the war. It was surrounded by factories. Next to the school stood Maynard's sweet factory, famous for making wine gums. The school had poor access – there were a few steps going out to the playground. Children in wheelchairs used a side entrance that only had one step. The school had four classes: one infant, two junior and a senior class. The headmistress had a voice like thunder. Everyone was frightened of her. She taught us singing once a week, which we all hated.

Mum wanted Mrs Collis's instructions to be obeyed: correct seating for me, and no writing. It wasn't long before my teachers complained about this, and Mrs

Collis reluctantly allowed me to use a very thick pencil. Eventually, I was treated at school by two successive physiotherapists, who had been trained by Mrs Collis. This pleased Mum very much.

Mum recognised three children at school who were outpatients with me in The Great Ormond Street Hospital. One of them, Sylvia, became a lifelong friend. Although Sylvia was a year older than me, we were in the same class. Sylvia's ingenuity in making the impossible possible appealed to me very much. She liked to help other people. Once, she wanted to help a neighbour who wasn't very well. She decided to make the old lady a cup of tea. The problem was how to take it to her. After much thought, Sylvia found a way. Having been able to walk when she was very young, Sylvia was quite steady on her feet. She made the tea in a small teapot to carry in her hand and put some milk in a small bottle with a tight lid. She put some sugar in a paper bag with a teaspoon, and put them all in a small case and took them to her neighbour. I was very impressed and started thinking of ways to do similar things. However, I had much work to do before I could match Sylvia's ingenuity. At home I volunteered to iron the handkerchiefs sitting down. I burnt my arm easily on the hot iron so I had to wear a cardigan for protection. I had to wait until I left school and was stronger on my feet before I managed to master tea-making. At first there was more tea on the table than in the teacup! I used a very small teapot.

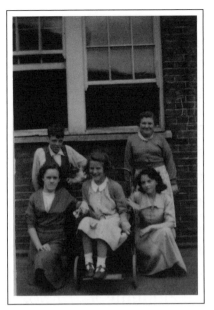

Sylvia, myself, Marjorie
and two friends at Vale
Road School.

When I started having domestic science lessons I often practised cooking on Saturdays, making cakes or pastries. Susan, a little girl Mum was looking after, and my sister were my helpers, fetching the ingredients, measuring out the flour and breaking the eggs. This venture was very successful, until one day my cakes didn't turn out quite right. My helpers had put wallpaper paste in the mixture instead of flour. After this disaster, I went off baking for while.

Sylvia and her friend, Marjorie, were quite mischievous. They were always getting me into trouble for giggling. My problem was I couldn't laugh quietly. Sylvia and Marjorie had nicknames for all the teachers. It was unheard of for children to know their teachers' first names, so my two friends made up their own names for our teachers. When I think of the humiliating way disabled children were treated in those days it's good to know there were some rebels about, like Sylvia and Marjorie.

Apart from children with physical disabilities such as cerebral palsy, tubercular hips, polio and limb amputations, some children had serious illnesses, like heart disease, making them appear blue. Some children spent most of the day lying down in the nurse's room after coming to school. One or two children died while I was there, which was very sad for me. It was my first experience of the death of someone close to me. Some children had deteriorating conditions, like muscular dystrophy, which was more common in boys. There were two brothers who had it. I always felt sad for the younger one as he must have realised his fate was going to be the same as his elder brother's.

When our strict headmistress retired, new teachers came and the quality of the lessons improved. Mr Ives, who taught the seniors art, became Headmaster. We noticed a great change in his character. Mr Ives was a very friendly teacher with a sense of humour, always making us laugh. The first thing he did when he became headmaster was to change his glasses, which made him look much more severe. He used to say, 'We don't want any passengers here,' and, 'The Lord helps those who help themselves.'

The seniors had a new teacher called Mr Wolfin who introduced us to drama. We started producing our own plays. Other new teachers joined the school and there was a general improvement in our curriculum. We were

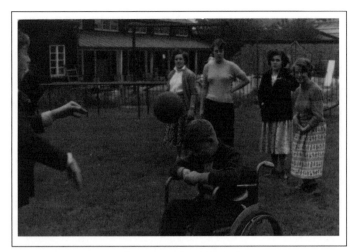

Playtime at Vale Road School.

very proud when a school uniform was introduced. The girls wore red and white candy-striped dresses and black blazers. The boys wore grey trousers and white shirts with their blazers. Our school badge was a serpent and an eagle, the sign of sickness.

Our school magazine was started, giving me a chance to develop my writing skills. I became joint editor. English Language and Literature became my best subjects. We started visiting places of historical interest: Hampton Court, the Houses of Parliament and museums. They provided plenty of material to write about in our magazine.

The school also adopted a ship belonging to the Royal Navy, called The Southern Cross. We regularly wrote to the crew. We visited the ship twice a year, once in the summer, and again for a Christmas party. These visits were enjoyed by everyone, and considered a very special treat. The ship was much larger than The Royal

49

Sovereign taking us to Southend for the day from Tower Pier, when I first started at the school. The Southern Cross looked very smart, giving the impression that the passengers were rich and famous.

Christmas was a good time to be in school. We had a big Christmas party, provided by the local Rotary Club, and presents which we were allowed to choose beforehand. Sometimes we went to the circus. It was very special time when we started producing our own entertainment for our parents. At first, we produced musical items. Then we did *A Christmas Carol*, just before I left school. It was an excellent production. I was the narrator.

In my final year at school, I learnt something new that provided me with a most valuable activity after leaving school. One day, my needlework teacher snatched the tea cosy I had been embroidering for ages in cross-stitch. She announced that she was going to teach me to make garments. She tried me on a sewing machine that was operated by turning the handle and I was delighted to find I could manage it and could even sew in a straight line.

In no time, I made a blouse. My teacher did the cutting out and pinning the pieces together. It was wonderful to be able to make something in such a short time. The worst thing was that I always needed someone at hand to help me when something went wrong with the sewing machine. The bobbin ran out of cotton or the needle became unthreaded. This was frustrating when working alone. Soon I was using an electric sewing machine and it was wonderful. I wanted to continue dressmaking after leaving school. My teacher asked if it was possible for me to come to her evening class. It was at least a couple of miles from home. Mum volunteered to push me to the class. Dad, who now had left the army and had a car, brought me home.

Soon I was making all my clothes. I was given my own electric sewing machine for my 21st birthday. The foot pedal was very small to find. Dad solved the problem by fixing a wooden gadget that provided a larger platform over the pedal, and this worked splendidly.

8
Rewarding Times

I had monthly check-ups from Mrs Collis in her clinic in Lambeth Hospital. She examined Margaret when she was only a few weeks old and found her to be physically perfect. At one of these appointments there was a problem getting transport home again. The clinic closed, and we were moved from department to department, whilst waiting for our transport. Margaret got very dirty playing on the floor in her blue woolly suit. We were tired and hungry. Mum had left a casserole cooking in a slow oven at home.

'Doesn't anyone care about me with my handicapped child and baby, stranded here far from home?' Mum pleaded with the hospital staff. They looked at her bewildered.

In desperation, Mum asked for directions to the police station. 'This is highly irregular. Are you telling the truth?' asked the police sergeant. Mum was beside herself. 'I am telling you. They're preparing beds for us for the night.' At last we were on our way home, thanks to the police. The casserole was burnt.

Mum complained profusely afterwards. There had been another patient called Ross attending the hospital that day who had cancelled his transport. On subsequent visits to Lambeth hospital, Mum was teased by the lady serving refreshments saying, 'Left anything in the oven today, Mrs Ross?'

To supplement the family income, Mum started looking after children at home. Suzanne, the first child in her care, was about Margaret's age. They were both toddlers. The first thing they did when they greeted each other every morning was to inspect each other's petticoats. Then came Susan. Mum named Susan 'Auntie Sue' because she was the eldest and came to us after school and on Saturdays. Susan was very good with the little ones. Robert joined the little group on Saturday mornings.

Mum cooked stews and rice puddings. She made jellies and banana custard for the children. The children ate well together and Mum encouraged them by getting everybody to clap for the first one who finished his or her meal. This was very popular with the children.

There was always plenty of washing up. Mrs Collis advised Mum to let me wash up sometimes to help me use my hands. Mum was horrified, anticipating the number of dishes I was likely to break. Mrs Collis suggested she use old crockery so that breakages wouldn't matter. She emphasised that my independence was the most important thing. So, every Saturday, sitting at the kitchen sink, I did the washing up. Of course there were lots of breakages. I was upset when I broke something. There were fewer accidents as time

I used a great deal of energy walking out and about. Mum encouraged me to drink plenty of milk and eat some chocolate every day. This did much to improve my stamina. Many people were praying for me at this time and I definitely felt their prayers were helping me. My appointments with Mrs Collis once a month at her clinic in Lambeth Hospital were extremely valuable. She instructed my physiotherapist at school about exercises I should do to help my walking.

In 1959 my friend Pat got married. I was a guest at her wedding. It was the first time I was able to walk around and mingle in a crowd. I wore a turquoise jersey suit and a white hat with a matching white handbag.

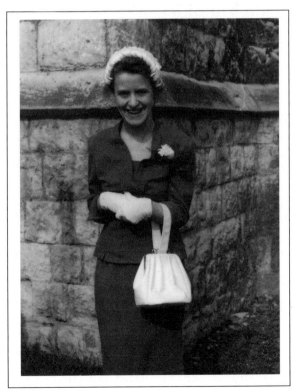

My outfit for Pat's wedding.

went on and I felt very useful. Doing the washing up greatly improved the co-ordination in my hands.

My progress continued. When I was thirteen, I no longer wore my skis. I could stand quite well and felt able to try to walk. I tried for the first time when my friend Margaret came to visit me. 'Go on then, have a go,' she smiled. I stood up, took a couple of steps, and then broke into a gallop across the sitting room. Margaret caught me and we collapsed on the floor in hysterics.

The next day, I decided to practise walking, taking a couple of steps at a time without falling over. I did this every day, starting off from the settee by the window and moving forward towards the door. After a few months, I walked to the kitchen and eventually managed to walk around my home. Independence, at last!

When I was fifteen I wanted to walk out-of-doors. I longed to be mobile. I had been given a self-propelling wheelchair and was disappointed that my arms were not strong enough to wheel myself. I waited a whole year for an adult's tricycle from a charity, only to find that I couldn't get on and off it myself. My feet had to be strapped onto the pedals. I soon realised I wouldn't be able to go anywhere on my own on the tricycle.

First, I challenged myself to walk across the lawn in front of my home to the seat at the edge of the pavement. I tried this one summer evening after school. It was a wonderful experience the first time I did it. I sat on the seat for ages. It was as if I was seeing everything for the first time: people, dogs, trees and cars. It was my first time out on my own two feet! A young man brought me an ice-cream cornet. He didn't realise the importance of the situation. Eating the ice cream was my little celebration for my great achievement.

It was a strange feeling, walking out of doors for the first time. I felt nervous about meeting people who knew me and had always seen me in a wheelchair. I felt very self-conscious. I wanted to walk further as my legs grew stronger, but I didn't feel ready to do this on my own. Fortunately, Margaret, now about four, was only too willing to come out with her big sister. Her endless chatter about fairies, witches and giants, as we walked along, was a perfect way to distract me from my self-consciousness. This was the start of many adventures together in the great outdoors. When I was able to walk further, and had enough confidence to go out by myself, I was glad of the low walls and seats scattered around the neighbourhood. I could sit on them and have a rest. Mum received many cruel comments about letting me walk out on my own. People had seen me fall over in the street and were concerned about me. Mum recognised my need for independence and wanted me to be prepared for the day when she would no longer be around to help me. Her confidence in me gave me the courage I needed. Dad, however, was uneasy about me walking outside on my own. Later, I found out that he followed me from a distance. If I had known this at the time I would have been rather cross with him.

Discovering how far I could walk and where I could walk to, when on holiday, was exciting and rewarding. I loved walking on the promenade of one of the beaches in Holyhead, feeling the sea breeze on my face and stopping to look at everything. I challenged myself to walk further to admire a different view. I could even walk to town from my grandmother's house and look at the shops. Once, I walked with my grandfather to a cousin's house. He looked so proud of me.

It was wonderful to be able to walk to church on Sunday morning. It took me about twenty minutes to get there, resting on a seat on the way. To be in fashion, I started wearing hats to match my dresses or coats. One of the chapel servants often whispered in my ear, 'I like your hat', which made me smile. Sometimes I got a lift home from his son in his red sports car.

9
Girl Guides

I hadn't been in the Vale Road School very long when my friends and I were invited to join the Girl Guides. It was a postal company, a special form of guiding. A scrapbook was sent to us once a month. It contained quizzes and items to tick off for roll-call and inspection. Some activities were written on coloured cards in envelopes, which were stuck on the pages of the book. It took about two hours to do everything. It must have taken a long time to prepare these books each month. There were labels with our names on so we could pass the books on to the next guide in the company. Most of my friends in school joined the Post-Guide Company.

Once a year, the Extension Guides, the name given to the disabled section, had a get-together in the summer. It gave us all the opportunity to sample camp food and singing around a real fire. We were also attached to a company near home. Going to a real meeting every week was the best kind of guiding. Two guides came to push me to the meeting in my wheelchair. The most attractive part of joining the organisation was wearing a special uniform. I was disappointed that my school didn't have a uniform – to wear one meant being part of the community. I was becoming aware how disability could exclude one from society by making one feel different.

Because of my disability I had to go to a different kind of school a long way from home and travel by coach. Consequently, local children didn't know anything about my school. My school friends lived too far away to exchange home visits. Joining the Girl Guides compensated for some of these differences.

Disabled guides did the same tests and badge work as everyone else. Alternative tests existed when disability made taking a test impossible.

I had to change my Guide Company after only having been there a very short time because we had moved home after my sister had been born. I found it much easier to integrate into the second Guide Company. In the first one I'd joined the girls were quite patronising. Ann, my patrol leader, was very tall and pretty. I'd found her rather overwhelming.

The new company was far more welcoming. Ethel Jones, our Guide Captain, was a sweet Scottish lady. She came to see me at home before I went to my first meeting. That first Guide meeting was quite something. The Poppy Patrol, my patrol, decided to quiz me. I could handle the general knowledge questions all right but not, 'What school do you go to?' I answered that I went to a special school by coach. Then came the next annoying question 'Do you go to school in the grey coach? We know someone who goes on that coach.' This made me very embarrassed and cross because it meant the coach taking the educationally subnormal children, as they were then called, to their special school. We often saw the grey coach on our school run. Mrs Baker, the coach escort, called it 'the Barmy Coach'. If I happened to see one of the Guides walking in the street I nearly fell off my seat trying to attract her attention to show her I was not on the grey coach. Thankfully, my new Guide friends decided I was just like them except for my disability. They said I would make a good member of their patrol.

One night, when I was going home, the two Guides who were usually very serious about pushing me home carefully, suddenly became giggly and started running with my wheelchair. The next thing I knew I had toppled out of my wheelchair. The shocked girls picked me up and put me back into it and continued to push me home in a more sombre mood. I was none the worse for the tumble and soon forgot all about it.

The following week when the same girls came for me they looked sheepishly at my mother who was helping me into my wheelchair. Then one of them spoke to me as we went along. 'Are you all right, Joan?' Looking puzzled, I replied, 'Yes, why?' One of the girls replied, 'We have been worrying all week about you after tipping you out of your chair. We thought your mother would give us a right telling off.' I laughed and said I had forgotten all about it. I hadn't even told Mum.

My mother and I often met people who imagined disabled children had learning difficulties. My Guide tests compensated for my not having exams at school. I had a great desire to prove myself. Learning something useful, and getting a badge for it, was a real feather in my cap.

I wore my navy Guide uniform for the first time when I was enrolled, having passed my 'Tenderfoot Test '. I had to learn the Guide Law, the Promise and Motto, the meaning of the Good Turn, the Salute and Handshake. I also learnt to do unusual things, like whistle signals, knots and tracking signs. It was difficult to learn the knots because I had to use my left hand. I am not left-handed but my left arm and leg are stronger than my right ones. Tracking signs and knots were useful in Guide camp. One tracking sign, a rectangle made from twigs, with five stones inside it and an arrow of twigs outside the rectangle, meant a letter was hidden five paces from the direction of the arrow. Knots were used for making furniture from twigs, such as shoe-racks.

Later, I took the second-class Guide test. The most exciting moment was lighting a campfire and cooking on it. I did this by giving instructions to another Guide. I also learnt some simple first-aid. Our knowledge of knots and tracking signs were put into practice in patrol activities in the summer months out-of-doors. It was great fun. I couldn't go camping with the Guides but once I was taken to spend the day with them in camp. I had a wonderful time. I watched them cook doughnuts and had a ride round the campsite in a trek cart.

Camping was the only activity I didn't participate in. I loved to help in the Scouts and Guides jumble sale. I usually helped on the bookstall. When there was a Church Bazaar I often sold coconut ice or was in charge of the 'Lucky Dip'.

In 1953, the Coronation Year, all the uniformed organisations belonging to the church put on a pageant in honour of the new Queen. I was Florence Nightingale's wounded soldier, wearing Dad's khaki army uniform. It was my first public performance on stage and it was wonderful.

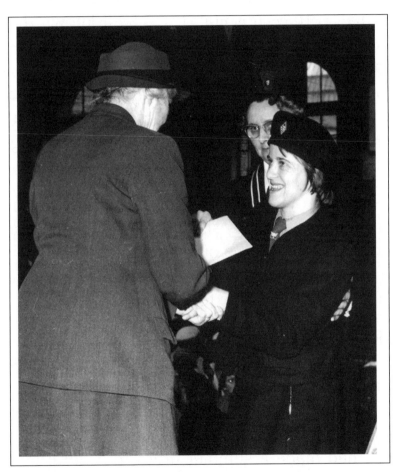

Being awarded a special award for fortitude by Lady Baden Powell, 1962.

10
The Rangers

I enjoyed being a Girl Guide very much. I looked forward to becoming a Ranger, which was the senior section of the Girl Guides for girls aged between 14 and 20. There were three sections: Land, Sea and Air Rangers.

I joined the Land Rangers with my friends, Maxine, Barbara and Frankie. Our uniform consisted of a grey shirt, with a navy scarf held together with a red leather ring we called a 'woggle', a navy skirt and forage-cap with a cloth Guide badge on it. It was a smart uniform. I felt very grown-up in the group. Some of the girls had

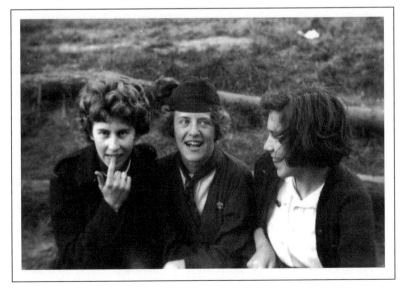

8th Crouch End Rangers and I, 1956.

already left school and were either working or attending college.

Renewing the Guide Promise was a grown-up affair. We promised to serve God and the Queen and keep the Guide Law. Rangers were also expected to serve the community. My disability was not seen as a barrier to serving others. I had always believed in God, although I hadn't yet developed a personal relationship with Him. I considered making this promise when I was the age of 14 as the first step to becoming a confirmed member of the Church. The 8th Crouch End Rangers were attached to the Moravian Church, the oldest protestant church in Europe. The followers of John Huss had founded it in 1457 in Bohemia, 60 years before Martin Luther started the great Protestant Reformation. I had experienced many kinds of worship before deciding to make the Moravian Church my spiritual home. The liturgical form of worship I enjoyed was similar to the Anglican Church where I had attended Sunday school. My first real opportunity to serve other people came when I was asked to help with a Brownie pack some way from home. I was beginning to take bus rides on my own. This would be good practice for me, using the buses. I only accepted the duty if I was able to make the journey myself. I managed this successfully. I came home with Tawny Owl in her bubble car. I loved helping the children with their badge work. They responded well to me.

The Ranger programme was varied and interesting. Once we did a motor mechanic's course. I couldn't see under the bonnet properly from my wheelchair. I had a good view of how to change a wheel. We were trained in first-aid by the Red Cross. We learnt how to make improvised splints and stretchers and how to stop severe bleeding. My little sister Margaret soon found out I was interested in first-aid. She came to me for advice saying, 'Joan, will you look at this scratch? Do you think it's going bad?' We both took these matters seriously. Once she came home with a nosebleed. She had walked into a lamp-post with her eyes shut. She wanted to know what it felt like to be blind.

After about a year in the 8th Crouch End Rangers, a new company was started for disabled girls in my school: The 1st Tottenham Land Ranger Unit. My friends, Sylvia, Sheila, Norma and I joined it. This group held monthly evening meetings at school. I was allowed to be a member of both companies. This had the advantage of enabling me to go to special camps and holidays. The local Rotarians provided us with transport. In between the meetings I enjoyed receiving plenty of post from the Guiders about forthcoming events. Letters posted in the morning reached me the same day. Soon we were off to our first camp. My doctor wouldn't allow me to sleep under canvas. Instead I slept on a camp bed in a shed with three walls, so I might as well have been under canvas. Sheila kept me company. One night there was a terrific thunderstorm. I'd never heard such loud thunder-claps before or seen such dramatic lightning. It cured me of being afraid of thunderstorms.

My new captain was quite prim and proper. She was a teacher in a girls' borstal. She was given some money towards our camp and bought us all artificial silk khaki pantaloons to wear in camp. She arranged a special weekend stay in an open borstal on a farm in Kent. I didn't know what to expect. A harsh prison-like system with plain food and water? It wasn't a bit like that. The girls were friendly and we had a lovely time. Afterwards, I enjoyed telling everyone I'd been to borstal.

In 1957, I had my first trip abroad. It cost £40. I had to save hard to raise the money for it. Four of us from my company went to Norway. A very special person ran these holidays. Her name was Miss Prentice and she made sure that there were no obstacles to having a good time. Sylvia and I were terrified of flying. At London Airport, I was sitting on the aircraft feeling scared. A woman, who was only three foot tall, looked at me and said, 'The Pilot has asked me to sit at the back of the plane to balance the weight.' I burst out laughing and forgot all about being nervous. Later, I learnt her name was Pip. She looked immaculate in her Guiders' uniform and carefully applied make-up. As we approached the coast of Norway at dawn, the twinkling lights on the numerous islands made it seem like fairyland.

Sylvia, Norma, Sheila and I were the youngest in the group. We shared a bedroom that was always in chaos. It was the first time we had had the responsibility for our belongings, and to be at the right place on time. It was a learning process in preparation for future independent holidays. Everything was a giggle to us.

On our second day we found a notice pinned to our bedroom door, saying: 'The Crazy Gang'. More giggles. It was good for me to be able to walk around the hotel, which was mostly made of wood. I walked a little outside, too.

One day Sylvia and I were walking towards our bedroom. Our footsteps made a lot of noise on the wooden floors. Suddenly we were aware of somebody else's footsteps. Miss Prentice was walking behind us imitating the way we walked. Of course we collapsed in hysterics. The hotel where we stayed outside Bergen had no lifts or ramps.

Those who couldn't walk were carried up and down the many steps. Miss Prentice carried some girls on her back!

One member of our group particularly impressed me. She lay flat on her back in a spinal carriage and looked at her surroundings through a mirror; she took photographs, holding her camera upside down. She must have had an amazing personality because she always had people around her laughing and joking. I was surprised to learn that she ran her own Brownie pack for non-disabled girls.

Three years later I went to Switzerland with the same group of Guides and Guiders. We stayed in Wilderswil outside Interlaken. We visited 'Our Chalet', an international centre for Guides. It was placed high up in the mountains. Guiders met us at the station and towed each wheelchair with ropes up the steep mountain paths. Another day, we went by train up to the snow-line and played snowballs. I had my first ride on a chairlift in Switzerland. Looking down on the twin lakes of Interlaken was breathtaking. However, I would have enjoyed the scenery much more if I hadn't been so scared of losing my shoes! My feet were precariously resting on the inadequate footrest.

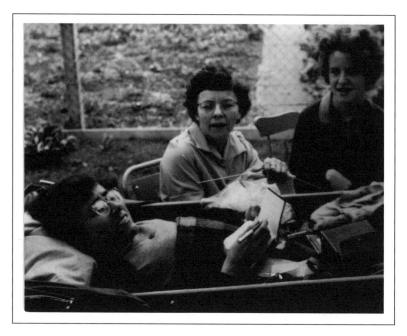

Guider in a spinal carriage.

I value my time as a Guide and Ranger. Guiding gave me self-esteem and gave me confidence to take my place in society. It prepared me for the disadvantages of disability in an able-bodied world. I was mixing with able-bodied girls of my own age as well as learning from my disabled peers.

11
Moving On

My childhood friend Margaret never did join the Guides. When she was 13, she told me she wanted a boyfriend. I started flirting with the boys at school a few years later. Margaret taught me the facts of life on Sunday evenings, mostly by telling me dirty jokes while our mothers were in church and once quoting from a pop song 'It only hurts for a little while'. It's strange that I was taught childcare in domestic science lessons but not how to make babies! Margaret married quite young and emigrated to Australia.

I dreaded leaving school. I became very depressed and was often reduced to tears. The normal leaving age in my school was 16 for physically disabled children. I was allowed to stay on until I was 18 because I was having physiotherapy at a crucial time, when I was learning to walk and making good progress.

Leaving school meant entering a world requiring ability, intelligence and strength. It seemed there were no allowances for imperfection. Disability was never featured in news bulletins, or seriously portrayed in any form of drama in the 1950s, only the odd joke about the 'Stupid Boy' or the 'Deaf Mute'. How could I make the grade in an able-bodied world where impairment implied weakness of body and mind? I was leaving a school where impairment was respected on the whole, and catered for. Outside would be very different. As I approached my 18th birthday, my mother attended meetings at school to discuss my future. I was not consulted. I could go to a residential training centre for disabled school-leavers, to be taught manual skills useful for employment. I wasn't impressed with this idea because I couldn't use my hands very well. My teachers were keen for me to go to the first grammar school, recently opened by the Spastics Society (now called Scope) for children with cerebral palsy. The Thomas Delarue School in Tunbridge Wells, Kent, was meant to be a centre of excellence, the first of its kind for disabled children in Britain. I would have loved to attend if it had been a day school. The final decision was made on the advice of Mrs Collis, who thought it inadvisable for me to study while I was learning to walk because I wouldn't be able to concentrate on both. I was very proud of my progress in walking. It was the most important thing to me. I agreed with Mrs Collis, who said she felt it would be more beneficial to attain my independence, rather than train to earn a living. Independence was a valuable goal to aim for.

My friend Sylvia left school before me. She found work in a factory making electrical parts for televisions. We met up at school once a month at Ranger meetings. It was good to have this opportunity of meeting up with school friends who had already left. It helped me immensely during this transition period. Being the middle of winter my first few months at home after leaving school were very bleak indeed, like the weather. I felt that I had been dumped on the scrap heap. Society had nothing to offer me, I was on my own now. Step by step I came to realise my destiny lay in my own hands. I thought about the value of my life. My difficult birth – I had had to be a resuscitated, nearly losing my life at six weeks from pneumonia. I knew my grandmother thought that I should have died at birth.

Doctors told Mum I would not grow up to recognise her. Well, they got that wrong! They also said I would never walk. I was beginning to walk.

On becoming a Christian I believed God had a purpose for me in life. I just had to find out what it was. Professional people didn't know everything. It was time to explore the possibilities awaiting me.

I had to do something to boost my morale. I decided to try to do something new each month, in addition to improving the distance I could walk. Useful things, like getting in and out of the bath, having a go at housework, washing-up and even tackling the weekly washing by hand. I felt more confident doing things when I was at home on my own. Other people made me nervous. Fortunately Mum found herself a part-time job so I was left alone for long periods.

* * * * * * * * * *

My confidence was growing because I was taking more responsibility for my own life. I was in control. One day, Mum said, 'I'm getting old now, I can't fight your battles anymore, it's up to you now.' Whatever path life

73

decided for me, I decided I was going to tackle it on my own two feet. I did not have to crawl. I would be knocking on many doors. Some would be slammed in my face before I found my small corner in life. Thanks to my parents and my wonderful, adventurous childhood, I was prepared to face life self-assured.

I consider myself very fortunate to have been old enough to understand the treatment that helped me so much. I was able to use my knowledge to help me overcome many physical difficulties, when trying to do something new. I think my parents became very proud of me and were justly so. I thank God for them. They have made me an independent person.

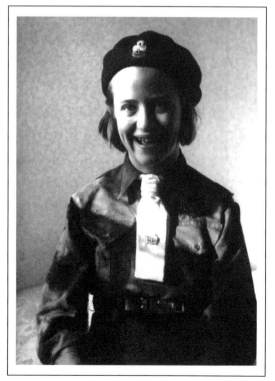

I join the Girl Guides, 1950.

12
Challenge

Leaving school in 1959 meant that my whole life was about to change. Born with cerebral palsy, I live in a body with limbs that are difficult to control. My speech is a little slurred. Yet I think like and have the same ambitions and dreams as an able-bodied person. It is very frustrating not to be accepted as such by society.

My social life began to be busy. I was in the Land Rangers and the senior section of the Girl Guides. I enjoyed discovering how to help other people and learning to serve the community. The same driver who took me to my Rangers' meetings volunteered to take me to an evening class for dressmaking. During my final year at school, I had developed an interest in this and was able to continue learning with the same teacher.

I joined a Bible class at the Mission Hall where I attended Sunday School. It was here that I met Brian. Brian was a year older than me. He was a student at the London School of Economics and had lodgings a few doors from where I lived. He started to push me in my wheelchair to classes. The class decided to join a Christian Youth Club in Muswell Hill. About twelve young people came along and offered to push me there and back every Saturday evening. As the weeks went on, fewer and fewer people turned up to push me. Finally Brian came for me by himself. I realised I had a crush on him. He had big brown eyes and black, wavy hair and spoke with a Lincolnshire accent. He looked after me with such care and enabled me to join in all the activities.

By constantly looking out of the window I knew the times Brian was likely to pass by. He often walked past with his landlady's ten-year old daughter, early in the evening on their way to the sweet shop. They did handstands on the grass in front of my living room window. I hid behind the curtain to watch them. Brian came home from college at about 3.30 p.m. He glanced over at my windows, looking for me. If I let him see me he ran to my front door. He stayed for ages, talking about all sorts of things.

He often greeted me, asking, 'What new thing have you learnt to do recently, Joan?' I tried to think of something impressive like, 'Oh, I threaded a needle today, it only took me thirty minutes.' Brian occupied most of my thoughts. Did he really fancy me? Lying in bed, I went over all the things he'd said to me, looking for clues to find out if he wanted to be my boyfriend. Mum showed concern. 'Brian's only being kind to you because you're disabled,' she said. I didn't want to hear this but I couldn't help taking notice. I was tormented by his attention. It was hard to distinguish between whether he was doing things for me because of my disability, or helping me because he liked me as a person. The last thing I wanted was to misinterpret his actions and cause myself extreme embarrassment. I was reluctant to discuss this with anybody as they might not understand.

The more we went out together, the more I felt we might kiss each other. However, I couldn't encourage him. One day I introduced Brian to a friend, Pauline, and she stole him from me. I felt sad for not having encouraged him more. However, maybe this hadn't been a good time to start a relationship. I needed to improve my mobility and independence. Brian and Pauline got engaged after a few months. Then they broke it off and Brian left the district.

Two things happened which gave me a bit of a boost. A new baby boy was born to the family in the flat above mine. His mother wasn't very well after the birth. Mum gave her quite a lot of support, so I got to know baby Simon quite well. When he was six months old his mum allowed me to push him around the grounds of our flats. Oh, what a joy it was the first time I pushed a baby's pram. I hadn't been able to push my sister's pram because I couldn't walk then. Another neighbour broke the rules about keeping pets and brought me her poodle to look after. Every time someone was due to come round from the Council, Mandy, the poodle, was brought down to us to be hidden.

After a while, Margaret, Mandy's owner, started work. Her dog barked and howled when left alone at home. So I became a paid poodle minder. My sister took her out for a walk when she came home from school. As time went on, I was able to take Mandy out. Another first for me. If I fell over on these walks, Mandy wouldn't let anyone else pick me up. She thought she was protecting me. When Simon was three his mum started work and his grandmother looked after him. Simon's tantrums were too much for his elderly granny so I became his carer with a little help from Mum. At first, Simon tested my patience by trying to do the most awful things he could think of. His tantrums didn't have the effect he'd hoped for because I just ignored them and they quickly ceased. Instead, he stood on a chair and yelled, 'Come on lions and tigers, and eat Joan all up!' I pretended to be frightened and it became a game. It was probably his way of protesting at being left by his mum. It was more acceptable behaviour than his tantrums, even though I was his victim!

Simon was fair-haired and had blue eyes. At four, he had become a charming little boy. Mum left our lunch for me to heat up but he wasn't keen on eating. I pressed his tummy to find a hole to fill with food, and it tricked him into eating his lunch. He proudly stuck his full tummy out after meals. I took Simon out shopping. When the shop assistant helped me put my shopping in my bag, and my change in my purse, I always said, 'Thank you very much. Goodbye.' And Simon also thanked her and said 'goodbye'.

When I became a Guider and had my own Brownie Pack Simon, was very helpful when I put on my uniform for Brownie meeting nights. Referring to my 'slippery hands', he buttoned up my shirt sleeves. Sitting astride my lap, he fastened my top button and pinned my brown owl badge on my tie. He concentrated so hard that his little tongue stuck out from the corner of his mouth.

Simon couldn't start school immediately after his fifth birthday because there was a shortage of teachers. Once, he heard me telling someone this. Afterwards, he paid me such a lovely compliment. He asked, 'Why don't you become a teacher, Joan, then I could start school and be in your class?' When Simon started school, his mum asked me to take him there on his first day. Then Mandy and I met him after school each day, and he stayed with me until his mum came home from work. I shall never underestimate the kindness of Simon's parents in entrusting me with their little son's care.

13
More Education Please

Encouraged by my physical progress and my success in voluntary work with children, I began to think about employment. First, I needed some 'O' levels. In the autumn of 1963, I was 24. I set off to enrol at the local adult education centre to study for the Royal Society of Arts English Language Course Stage One. A television soap called *Crossroads* had started and my sister, Margaret, was watching it. It began just as I was leaving home to sign up for the course. I walked to the rhythm of the signature tune in my head. My legs felt very heavy as I walked up the pleasant pathway to the school built on the playing fields. I was so nervous.

I walked into the crowded hall. There were men and women seated by desks with the name of the subject on card. Queues were forming. I joined one of them. Someone offered me a chair to sit on and wait my turn. Soon, it was over. I had done it. Nobody asked, 'What about your disability?' or, 'How will you manage the writing?'

Walking home again was so different – I was so excited.

I knew that English language was a good subject for me to start with. I enjoyed writing. To build up my confidence I chose to start with the basics. I couldn't wait for the class to begin. The next week I set off for my class. As I walked towards the school I felt very apprehensive. Would I be able to keep up with the rest of the class? Would I find the work too hard? I was disappointed to find the lecturer was absent. He had left some written work for us to do. I started working through it as quickly as I could. Half way through the evening there was a break for tea or coffee. I carried on working in case I didn't finish in time. When it was time to hand in our work I looked at my handwriting and wondered what the lecturer would think of my strange scrawl. I decided to write on the bottom of the page, 'Please note I am a spastic.' In the 1960s the word 'spastic' was not used to verbally abuse people. I was grateful for the word 'spastic'. People understood that word. It meant that somebody couldn't use their limbs properly and would explain the wobbly writing. The following week, the lecturer walked into the classroom and gave me a friendly smile and I knew everything would be all right.

I wrote quite a few letters. It was the only way of communicating with people. There was no telephone at home. Once I tried to phone from a public call box. I was almost connected but then I dropped the receiver and broke part of the mouthpiece. I felt dreadful and it was a long time before I ventured near a phone box again. Writing in good English became a valuable tool in my life.

I had the same lecturer throughout my English language course. Mr Lamb was kind and did much to build my confidence. He taught at the local junior school. My sister knew him. Mr Lamb came from Durham and had a warm northern accent. He loved reading and I often saw him in the local library. Mr Lamb often mentioned his Russian wife in class and his two daughters who were close to my sister's age.

I sat my first exam a year later and passed. Oh what excitement! I was allowed 30 minutes extra time in consideration of my difficulty in writing. One year later I took the R.S.A. Stage Two. Then I had the confidence to sit my first G.C.E. 'O' level.

At first, I was only given ten minutes extra time. I was shocked. This was ridiculous. How could the examining board have so little understanding of disability? Possibly, it was unusual to have disabled students sitting exams. I sought the help of the North London Spastics' Association (later renamed, North London Cerebral Palsy Association) to negotiate for extra time and was given an extra 30 minutes.

I was a little self-conscious about studying for 'O' levels in my early 20s. Due to a shortage of teachers in the 1960s daytime classes in G.C.E. 'O' levels for women were started in my area. I happily integrated into this group. I was attending an English Literature class at Southgate Technical College. The journey to classes, taking two to three buses, was often an adventurous and hair-raising experience.

I needed a carbon copy of someone's notes. I decided to ask Irene because she looked so kind. 'Please may I have a copy of your notes?' I asked, flinging some carbon and paper in her direction. Despite scaring the life out of her, she said yes, and we became very close friends. Irene had a lovely Liverpool accent. A good sense of humour matched her cheeky elfish face. Her little boy had just started school and she had a daughter in the Juniors. Her family, including her husband, gave her a hard time because she was studying.

I was very fortunate in gaining two 'O' levels in my own handwriting with so little extra time. The faster I wrote the more illegible my writing became. My luck changed when I sat the geography exam. After failing it twice it was realised I would never pass because I couldn't use a ruler. I even tried using a special heavy ruler. The compulsory question requiring a map drawn to scale gained half the exam marks. I was bitterly disappointed. I loved geography.

In the time it took me to pass two 'O' levels the other women in my class had passed five 'O' levels in one go and they all went on to teacher training college. Irene also went on to a teacher training course. After qualifying she was offered a position as head of a nursery school. Sadly, within a few days of telephoning me, she had a massive brain haemorrhage and wasn't able to use her qualification as she would have wished. Irene is such a lovely person and she didn't deserve such bad luck. We are still good friends.

I eventually abandoned the carbon paper for a large tape recorder. Carried in a small holdall, it often tumbled off the bus in front of me as I alighted. I was always pleased when the bus drew near enough to the kerb, to make it easier to step on or off. Once, when I got off a bus, and inwardly congratulated myself on a perfect landing, someone called, 'You shouldn't be out on your own.' I turned and saw a woman, glaring at me with her hands on her hips. Without a word to her, inwardly chuckling, I walked to my class.

Failing other exams beside geography didn't deter me from trying again because my tutors were so encouraging. I enrolled for the same courses again. However, one tutor, who hadn't taught me, said,' Are you here again?' with a look that implied that I was wasting my time.

One day, a lecturer asked me if I could type or dictate my exam answers. She thought the reason for failing my exams was due to my handwriting. I wasn't confident enough to dictate to anyone. I had tried manual typewriters before; the keys were too heavy. The ribbons often fell out and became tangled. I had heard about electric typewriters. I hired one for a few days, and found I could type using a pencil with a rubber on it. So, I could type with one finger on one hand. The local cerebral palsy association bought me a lovely portable electric typewriter. I had three months to learn how to use it. I worked through old exam papers before my exams trying to improve my speed. I still needed extra time. No examining board allowed me more than

30 minutes. A few months later, I gained an 'O' level in history, and an 'A' level in English. My persistence had paid off. Between 1968 and 1975, I gained 5 'O' levels - English language, English literature, history, sociology and British Constitution. I also passed English and sociology at 'A' level, thanks to my electric typewriter. Regretfully, I never succeeded in Geography.

14
My Own Brownie Pack

When I was a Ranger I was asked if I would like to help guide the Brownies, as some of my friends were helping with the Brownies and Cubs. I was delighted. The pack meetings were some distance away. I didn't want my Mum to push me there in my chair. I was just starting to ride on buses on my own. I thought this would be a great opportunity to get used to making regular bus journeys to build up my confidence. I was promised a lift home.

I was fascinated with the games and activities planned for girls between 7 and 11 years old. Many were designed as a fun way of learning. I thought of more activities to do with Brownies. I taught small groups of children their knots and first-aid. They accepted my clumsy movements and were eager to help me.

A year later, the Brownie Guider in my Church pack resigned. I desperately wanted to take her place. I didn't offer for fear of being rejected. To my surprise, the District Commissioner asked me if I would like to take over the Brownie pack. I was over the moon. There were certain conditions as leader that I readily accepted. The maximum number of girls in my pack must be restricted to eighteen instead of twenty-four, and I must always have two people helping me.

When I took over, my sister was one of the older Brownies. Many of her friends were regular visitors at home. This had its disadvantages. If I did anything wrong I'd hear about it when I came home, for example, 'You forgot to give Jane her cook's badge.'

I went on weekend residential training courses for Brownie Guiders. One trainer was HRH Princess Anne's Brownie Guider. I thoroughly enjoyed these courses. I couldn't wait to try out the things I'd learnt. After a while, the District Commissioner came and watched me take a few meetings and asked a few questions before awarding me a Guiders' warrant.

Every meeting began with 'Brownie Ring.' The Brownies danced around the toadstool singing 'We're the Brownies here's our aim. Lend a hand and play the game.' I managed to dance round the toadstool with the Brownies. We danced slowly for my benefit. The Brownies didn't seem to mind this. I think it was important for me to join in the ceremony.

The Pack was divided into three groups called 'Sixes' that were named after Fairies: Elves, Sprites and Gnomes. They sang their own little songs as they danced round the toadstool. Elves: 'This is what we do as elves, think of others not ourselves.' Sprites: 'Here we come, the sprightly Sprites, helping others throughout the night.' Gnomes: 'Here we come, the laughing gnomes, helping mothers in their homes.' Each 'Six' had a leader called a 'Sixer' and a second in command called a 'Seconder'. The older Brownies were appointed as leaders. While we were standing round the toadstool I gave out badges, announced notices, inspected uniforms and enrolled Brownies.

We also sat round the toadstool for a story at the end of the meeting. I chose not to read from a book. Instead I made up a story. Very often I couldn't finish the story in time to close the meeting and had to continue it the next week. One week a Brownie came to the meeting with her face all swollen after having a tooth out. 'Why didn't you stay home tonight Susan?' I said, a little concerned to see her poor swollen face. 'Oh no, Brown Owl, I couldn't do that. I wanted to hear the end of your story.' I was very touched at this compliment.

To compensate for my disability, I had to invent different ways of doing things. I couldn't hold semaphore flags so I used cards with the flags drawn on them instead. I couldn't skip with a rope but I knew what I wanted the girls to achieve: shoulders back, chin up, toes together, and arms horizontal! Many Brownies got through their first class test and gained a sleeve full of interest badges. After a Brownie made her promise before being enrolled, my assistant guider 'Snowy Owl' pinned the badge on her tie on my behalf, as I couldn't do it.

I hope I was teaching these children to have a positive attitude towards disability, just as I had to find different ways of doing things with them. They instinctively adjusted to my disability. They readily helped me get up when I fell over. Before the invention of plastic straws, they held my drinks for me.

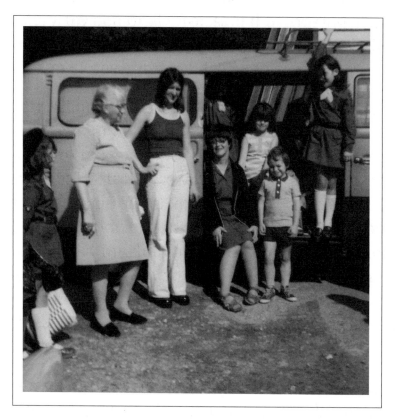

My Brownie pack on holiday, 1972.

I hadn't had the pack very long when, in 1962, Middlesex East County Guides held a rally in Alexandra Palace. Lady Olave Baden Powell, The Chief Guide, attended it. During the afternoon, my name was called and I was escorted onto the platform to receive a special award for fortitude from the Chief Guide. There was a deafening cheer in the great hall. Next week, my photo with Olave Baden Powell was in the local paper.

I was very surprised to receive this award so soon after taking over the Brownie pack as I didn't think I'd earned it yet. However, I stayed with the pack for fifteen years. At the same time I became Assistant Guider and later Captain in the Ranger Company of teenage girls with a disability, which was attached to my old school.

Little girls in the 1960s were not into fashion or pop. They liked to please. Brownies were fascinated with the idea of doing nice things for their adult relations. The Brownie motto was 'lend a hand'. I explained the motto to new recruits as follows: 'Suppose it starts raining and Mummy has some washing drying on the line. If you bring the washing in, this helps Mummy.' This made the Brownies' faces light up.

When I first took over I walked to the meetings. I visited the Brownies' parents at home. It was very tiring but necessary. I was determined to ensure my Brownies didn't lose out by having a disabled leader. We had a couple of outings every summer. Over the years, we visited many places of interest in London: the zoo, the Planetarium, the Science Museum, RoSPA House and many other places. I had two children with mobility problems in the pack, Jane and Fiona. They both attended local schools and joined in everything. Jane always made for the front seat of the bus on our outings. They all loved having picnics. Once, a Brownie fell in the paddling pool and got soaked. I was partly prepared for accidents, carrying a first-aid kit and a spare uniform dress. My assistant, Snowy Owl asked, 'Is anyone wearing two pairs of knickers? In a flash a child stepped forward, took her top pair of pants off and said, 'Here you are Brown Owl.'

Before going on an outing, I often smiled as I approached the Church Hall. A good number were always early with their huge bags of food and bottles of pop. Some were already eating. I was never late.

On winter evenings, it was quite difficult to open up the hall for pack meetings. The church and hall were on a main road positioned on a service road. The hall was at the back of the church with a path leading to it from the side. It was very dark and creepy accessing the hall on winter evenings. I could hardly see the keyhole of the hall door. Inside, I had to find the key on a chain on the wall and place it in two different slots to switch on the light in the lobby and the outside light for the footpath. It was very hard for me. I should have asked the church committee to put in proper light switches but I was too independent. In spring and summer I wasn't short of help. Someone was always waiting at the gate to say, 'Hello Brown Owl, can I take your bag?'

There is a difference between meetings held in summer and those held in winter. Before central heating was installed we did lots of running around games to keep warm and let off steam. Visitors often found that my meetings were very quiet compared with other Brownie pack meetings. As I couldn't shout very loudly the child nearest to me repeated my instructions to the others: 'Brown Owl says stand in a circle.' In summer games were played outside on the church lawn. It gave the children an opportunity to learn about nature.

I usually carried many items in my bag to use in the Brownie meetings. Apart from my register and quiz cards that I had prepared during the week I also borrowed things from home, anything from a kitchen knife to a pillowcase. Such were the variety of activities each week. In fact the activities of the Brownies spilled into my home so often that Mum said, 'I feel like wearing a Brownie uniform myself.'

In my final few years with the Brownies I took them on Pack Holidays. Having passed my test for the special warrant I was assisted by some very experienced Guiders, but definitely felt in control and responsible for the holiday activities. The holidays usually had a theme. One year it was a voyage on ship and we did a special ceremony involving King Neptune ducking the girls in water to mark 'The crossing of the Equator'.

15
Bus Rides

When I first started going on a bus I was quite nervous. I comforted myself, thinking, 'There's bound to be somebody on the bus that knows me.' I had lived in the same area for so long. Getting on and off the bus and sitting down before the bus moved off was the most dangerous part of the journey. I often felt a hand supporting me from behind getting on and off the bus. I very rarely saw whom the hand belonged to but I always said, 'Thank you,' anyway. It was my guardian angel looking after me. I always reassured people about my guardian angel when telling them about my adventures on buses. The bus drivers got to know me well. As I approached the bus stop they often gestured to me asking me if I was getting on the bus. If I wasn't I shook my head to indicate no.

Once something went horribly wrong as I approached the bus. It was about to move off. I was the only one getting on. The driver had seen me but the conductor saw me only after ringing the bell signalling the driver to move off. He rang the bell again to tell the driver not to move off. I had one foot on the step and was holding the handrail but the bus moved off before I was properly on board. I instinctively hung on to the rail for dear life and was dragged along for what seemed like a few yards before I let go falling back hitting my head on the kerb. It was a very frightening experience. People rushed to my assistance, half carrying me into Boots the chemist. I was bleeding from the back of my head.

A woman administered some first-aid while I waited for an ambulance. When it came I asked to be taken to the small cottage hospital. I was well-known there, a regular visitor to the small casualty department. I was always cutting myself on broken glass and china when doing the washing up. The sister in charge used to come into the waiting room and say, 'Anyone for casualty.' I put my hand up shyly and she burst out laughing, 'Oh no, not you again Joan.'

On the day of my accident it must have been late afternoon. The casualty sister wasn't there. Instead the old matron took charge of my treatment. She knew me well too. She called a doctor to stitch me up and stayed with me until I was able to go home.

It took a long time to get over this terrible accident. I lost my nerve and wouldn't go on any more bus rides for a whole year. I missed going by bus because I was now limited as to where I could go. After a year I plucked up the courage to try once again to take a bus ride. I had made a summer dress in a floral material of black with bright yellow flowers. I wanted a hat to match so I waited for the day when I felt brave enough to try to get on the bus again to visit Wilson's Store in Crouch End. It was just two stops. Feeling a little shaky I climbed on the bus and sat down. Soon I was in

Crouch End and I carefully alighted off the bus. 'Yippee, I've done it!' I said inwardly. It felt wonderful. I went into Wilson's and took my time choosing a hat. I found one that I liked very much and made my way back to the bus stop to take me home. Everything went well and before I knew it I was back safely at home again. I felt wonderful, I just wanted to get on a bus again and do it all over again!

I was encouraged by my successful bus ride and overcoming my fears of further accidents. I soon had plenty of ideas of places I would like to go to by bus. I found bus maps very useful when I started travelling by public transport again. It was very exciting to plan my journeys. I joined the Church study group in the '60s. The topic was 'Good Neighbours'. There were several tasks to choose from, relating to this topic. The most appealing to me was a visit to a law court. I decided to go to the top, The Old Bailey. I planned my journey and was very excited when the great day arrived. However, I woke to find a gale force wind blowing. I'd have difficulty walking in such windy conditions. I discussed it with Mum over breakfast, and then decided perhaps it would be better if I went to the Highgate Magistrates' Court instead.

I found my way to the court but it was closed. I decided that, since I had got this far safely I might as well go to the Old Bailey. I caught the bus from Highgate. When I reached Holborn Viaduct, the wind was so strong I could hardly stand up. I needed to cross the road. I noticed an elderly gentleman waiting to cross over too.

I asked, 'Please may I hold on to your arm to cross the road?' The gentleman nodded and we crossed the road together. I soon found myself outside the Old Bailey. I proudly approached the policeman at the entrance. 'Please may I come and listen to one of the court cases?' The policeman looked thoughtfully before replying, 'I can take you to Court No 1, on the top floor, if you can climb the stairs.' I nodded that I could.

Sitting in court, I was so overwhelmed that I had actually made it that I couldn't concentrate on the first case. I settled down and tried to understand it. I soon realised the person was on trial for stealing and murder. An elderly couple had been robbed in their home. The wife was found dead from stab wounds and the husband died later in hospital. He had also been stabbed. Two hundred pounds in cash had been taken and some jewellery was also missing. The accused had been arrested six months later.

The accused was Scottish and spoke with a strong dialect. 'Maybe ah goat oaf at the same bus stoap as the auld doll, but ah didnae fallay her hame.' Someone in court said, 'My lord, the witness said, "Maybe I got off at the same bus stop as the old lady, but I didn't follow her home."' I found it all very fascinating because I was studying for my GCE 'O' level at the time and appreciated the importance of clarity in language. I smiled to myself, hearing the old lady referred to as 'doll', this was my special pet name for Mum these days, especially when I wanted to put her in a good mood. I stayed in court about an hour and a half, before making my way home. I stopped in a cafe in Fleet Street for a cup of tea before catching the bus home, feeling very pleased with myself.

16
I Want to Learn to Drive

Two of my friends had been issued with invalid cars, which enabled them to drive to their jobs as typists. They both had polio. Linda couldn't walk at all and Janet couldn't travel on public transport.

Invalid cars were supplied and maintained by the Ministry of Health. They were made of fibreglass. Some had a canvas roof and were painted pale blue. These three-wheelers only had one seat for the driver and could easily topple over. Strong winds could blow them off-course. They were powered by petrol or batteries. The electric version only did 10 m.p.h. The Ministry gave a stringent medical to applicants, and paid for three driving lessons soon after the vehicle was delivered.

Much as I enjoyed travelling by bus, it was beginning to cause pain in my muscles and tendons. Seeing the extra glow in my friends' faces when they mentioned their cars, I decided to apply for one too. Mum wasn't happy at the suggestion. She'd never opposed any of my ventures before. 'What about the way you jump when you are in Dad's car and you think someone's going to hit us?' she asked. She jumped too. I gave her comment serious thought. Then I decided that I felt nervous travelling with Dad because I wasn't in control of the vehicle or didn't have a driver's view of the road. So I applied for a car.

I attended a medical at the Ministry of Health office in Euston Road, London. I obeyed the doctor's instructions. 'Squeeze my hand. Press on my arm.' I felt confident but not for long. He asked me to pick up a pin from a polished table. I tried but it was impossible. 'That's it,' I thought, 'I've failed, I won't get a car.' I went home feeling deflated.

Eventually, I had an appointment at a Ministry garage where invalid cars were serviced and repaired. 'I'd better not mess this up!' I thought. I sat in a three-wheeled vehicle and was pushed around a yard by some men. I had to apply the brakes by depressing the 'T' bar. This made the car swerve slightly to the right.

Incredibly, this mini-assessment was sufficient to allow me a battery-powered invalid car that would do 10 m.p.h. I was delighted. I couldn't have a petrol car with a maximum speed of 50 m.p.h., as I couldn't manage the gears. The car had to be garaged with access to electricity to charge it. Fortunately, a garage near my home became vacant and I took it over. I had to apply to the council to install an electric socket in the garage. It took a year to get everything in place before the car was delivered.

My car arrived in December 1971. I posted the required document to obtain road tax for it. My excitement grew in anticipation of soon being able to drive. On January 1st 1972, the postal workers went on strike. This lasted until the second week of March. Waiting for the road tax to arrive was unbearable.

At last the great day came for my first driving lesson. An instructor arrived from the British School of Motoring. He was a very small man, and had to be or he couldn't have fitted into my car! I got into it, and he squeezed in beside me looking very uncomfortable. After a few words of introduction, I was told to turn on the ignition. Nothing happened. After being left stationary for so long in the coldest time of year, the batteries had given up their will to live. I was very disappointed. The instructor and I parted company, planning to meet again when the car was working.

A few days later, I was ready for my second lesson. Unfortunately, it was booked for 6.30 p.m. in the middle of rush-hour. At last the instructor arrived and this time the car actually moved. The lesson consisted of driving around the block several times. All I had to do was to follow my instructor's commands. 'Signal left, turn left. Stop.' We went round the block again making right turns. The lesson was over very quickly. I was exhausted.

A few days later I had my second lesson and went through the same process, except this time I drove my car into the garage. At the end of the lesson, the instructor told me my driving course was finished. 'It's up to you now,' he said, 'I've taught you all you need to know.' He used a derogatory tone of voice that implied that if I couldn't drive this simple vehicle I must be very stupid.

Eventually, I would take a motorcyclist's driving test. However, there was no hurry to do this now. I could keep my 'L' plates on for as long as I wished. I felt safer this way, assuming drivers would be more considerate. It was very important for me to be able to drive my car in and out of the garage. I discussed this with Irene, a student in my English literature class, the same friend who'd let me have a carbon copy of her notes. We'd become good friends. She offered to come along and give me moral support while I practised driving in and out of the garage. I reversed the car out successfully. Driving it in again was a little more difficult. I had to get the car up a steep camber and it just wouldn't go. Then suddenly it shot forwards and hit the garage door! Oh dear, there was a horrible crack on the left side of the car bonnet. We both turned pale. Somehow, I managed to get the obstinate car back into the garage. My friend and I went sorrowfully back indoors to have a soothing cup of tea. I felt demoralised. I had to report the accident to the Ministry of Health and wait a few weeks for the car to be repaired.

The vehicle was driven with the same controls as a motorbike. It had a throttle on a 'T' bar, which served as a steering column. To accelerate I turned the throttle away from me. To slow down I turned it towards me. While waiting for the car to be mended, I considered how I could gain better control of it. I thought about my earlier medical treatment in childhood that had got me standing and walking by using the intelligent part of my brain to control my limbs. This method eventually created patterns in my brain, giving me more control of my limbs. I tried the same technique to gain control of the throttle. I found something of the same thickness and practised turning it backwards and forwards at different speeds in the safety of my home. A large plank was attached to the foot brake, so I had no trouble applying the brake in an emergency. To gain proper control I practised pressing my foot indoors on a big sponge. When I drove again, I found a marked improvement in using the controls.

I was very nervous about driving again. When my church minister visited me and heard my sad story, he offered to help by driving behind me round Crouch End. He came a few days later and it was very reassuring. My confidence grew as I practised driving. We arranged to stop occasionally to discuss my progress and soon I was ready to go out on my own.

Driving an electric car meant there was always a risk of breaking down with a flat battery. I had to avoid hills. I picked a special route to my classes at the technical college but there was one hill I couldn't avoid. I sometimes broke down on it and had to continue my journey home by bus. Driving at 10 m.p.h. was quite hazardous. Drivers hooted me as they overtook me. 'Yes, Mum, I did jump,' I admitted. At first I thought that drivers were criticising my driving and did not realise that they were signalling to pass me. I managed to avoid any accidents. A friend who often saw me when she went by bus said, 'Joan, I saw a huge traffic jam the other day, and guess who was at the head of it? It was your car holding everyone up!' I could never overtake anything. Once I tried to overtake a milk float but we just ran side-by-side, and I had to drop behind again. Another day I was excited to see mounted police ahead of me. 'I wonder if I can overtake them!' I thought as I was getting near them, and yes, I did pass them! I was elated and told everybody.

Several years later cars with automatic transmission came into mass production, including invalid cars. I applied for one. It was still made of blue fibreglass with three wheels. It had a small luggage space behind my seat and a folding one beside me that was not meant for passengers. It was there to slide onto to reach the door. I had three more driving lessons. The car's maximum speed was 50 m.p.h. The instructor looked far more comfortable sitting beside me on the bench in this car than my previous instructor had been in my other car. The first thing he did was to put a notice on the back car window saying: 'Please keep your distance.' This made me feel much safer and I enjoyed many years driving this car. Learning to drive was surely one of the best things to happen to me.

17
Going on Holiday by Car

I wanted to go on a holiday, and I wanted to travel by car. I approached Janet who also had an invalid car. She was all for it. I suggested going to the guesthouse in Westgate-on-Sea, Kent where we once stayed with the Rangers. Janet liked my suggestion. It required a great deal of planning in order to reassure our families and ourselves that we could do it. The journey was 82 miles from home. The best option was to travel on the A2 from the Blackwall Tunnel.

First we tried some long journeys. I suggested going to Southend for the day to visit my first Ranger captain who now lived in Shoeburyness. Stopping on the way, Janet and I joined the AA. Now we were fully prepared for any emergency. The journey was trouble free. I felt so proud when parked beside Janet's car on the seafront in Southend before visiting my Ranger captain. I didn't tell her in advance of our visit in case we didn't make it. She looked very shocked when she saw us on her doorstep.

She didn't approve of our adventure. 'You girls have travelled on an extremely busy, treacherous road,' she said, as she served us with tea and sandwiches. A few days later I had a further 'ticking off' in a letter. It was best not to tell her what the final goal was to be. A holiday in our own cars!

Janet chose Syon Park for our second outing. As usual traffic on the North Circular Road was heavy. I had planned the route so I led in front. Cars overtook us and it was difficult to stay behind each other. Separated by cars and lorries; losing sight of each other several times. I wished we had 'walkie talkie' radios to keep in touch. When I reached the car park in Syon Park, there was no sign of Janet. She came after a while, having taken a wrong turn. Janet had brought her wheelchair. We took it in turns to wheel each other round the park. Another successful trip.

Finally, my sister and her husband offered to take me to Westgate for the day in their car. This would enable me to familiarise myself with the route to Westgate -on-Sea. Preparations complete, we could now look forward to a great holiday.

Westgate-on-Sea is a very pretty area, quieter than Margate, about two miles along the coast. Our guest-house, 'Ocean Swell', was on the sea front. The guests were mainly disabled. It had a great family atmosphere. Janet and I shared a bedroom overlooking the seafront, something we very much appreciated. It took us five hours to drive there. We usually stopped every two hours on the way. Janet sat in my car for a chat and a cup of tea or coffee made from flasks of boiling water. How we enjoyed these breaks. It was lonely driving on our own. We needed to exchange comments on the thoughtless drivers who cut us up on the road. I also found that holding the throttle for too long caused pins and needles in my hand. I welcomed the stop to revive my circulation again.

Mr and Mrs Camp ran the guesthouse. It had a bar; Friday night was party night. When the weather was bad Mrs Camp often played the piano for a singsong. Janet and I explored the area visiting Canterbury, Herne Bay and Ramsgate. We also visited some very pretty villages. It was possible to reach the sandy beach at Westgate. I bought folding chairs that fitted in my car for Janet and me to sit on the beach. We loved coming to Westgate. It was only possible to drive on the motorway when it wasn't windy. When we started to go to other places for our holidays we still came back to Westgate-on-Sea at Easter.

One Easter, on the Good Friday, I woke up to find it was snowing. 'You will have to cancel your trip because of the weather.' Dad warned me. I wasn't sure as the snow didn't seem to be settling. I rang Janet to ask what she thought. We decided to go and met in Tottenham early. On reaching Kent the weather improved and we arrived in sunny Westgate about 12.30pm. After resting on our beds for a couple of hours Janet got up first and looked out of the window just in time to see a couple of invalid cars arrive. I joined her at the window. We both got very excited as we had always been the only ones with invalid cars. Within an hour the car park had a dozen or so invalid cars. Members of The Disabled Drivers' Club had come there for the weekend. We had a fantastic time with them. The next day everyone went out in convoy to Wickhambreux, a small picturesque village. You should have seen the look on people's faces as we drove down the country lanes. It must have looked like a 'Martian Invasion'.

One of the members, John, fascinated me by his agility. Having no use in his legs he swung around from chair to chair, using his arms, and up onto the bar to order his beer. Out in the car park he darted around in his wheelchair, helping everyone. It was an unforgettable weekend.

In 1976, Janet and I decided to try and have a holiday in the Isle of Wight. It took a great deal of planning.

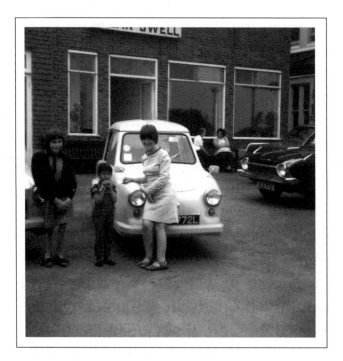

First holidays by car, 1972.

First, checking the distance from London to the ferry port in Lymington to ensure we caught the ferry on time and second, finding suitable, affordable accommodation. I learnt from Dad the importance of estimating the distances en route and budgeting for the cost of the holiday. There were no such thing as credit cards then!

In the 1960s, Dad took Mum, Margaret and me all over Europe by car. I always navigated for him. Unlike Janet and myself, Dad didn't book the accommodation in advance. On our travels through Europe we stayed at a different 'pension' each night, in small villages in France, Belgium and Germany. Margaret and Dad walked round the little villages. We had to stay somewhere approved by my fussy little sister! We spent some lovely holidays in Austria, Yugoslavia and Italy.

We travelled in convoy as usual, making several stops along the way using the M3 motorway. Our cars on motorways seemed to irritate other motorists. On entering a motorway, a large notice displayed a list of certain vehicles prohibited using it. It included invalid carriages. Unfortunately, motorists thought we were driving these and gave us a hard time. On our way to the Isle of Wight, a lorry driver persistently flashed his lights, hooted and signalled me to pull up on the hard shoulder so that he could tell me to leave the motorway, or he would report us to the police.

'We are not driving invalid carriages,' I explained, waving an article clarifying the difference between the two kinds of vehicles, published by the Disabled Drivers' Association. 'Invalid carriages are hand propelled and have a maximum speed of 10 m.p.h. We are driving petrol invalid cars with a maximum speed of 50 m.p.h.' 'I'm still reporting you both,' he grunted. We never saw him again and continued our journey. He put us in great danger, making us stop on the hard shoulder.

1979 is memorable as being a very hot summer. The grass everywhere was parched. I wore sandals for the first time. They actually stayed on my feet and I walked quite well in them. Freshwater Bay is a quiet seaside town and not too commercialised. During our week's stay we were able to explore the whole island. Everywhere was easy to reach even though most of the roads were narrow and we couldn't drive very fast. We visited places such as Osbourne House, Carrisbrooke Castle and East and West Cowes. Janet and I visited some nature reserves taking our time walking around looking at everything spending the whole day at one place.

Having found a car park on the high cliff overlooking the bay close to Freshwater, we spent the evenings here after dinner, watching the sun going down, sipping cups of tea bought from a nearby kiosk.

18
In Pursuit of a Teaching Career

I felt very proud of having gained five 'O' levels and an A-level in English. My success with my Brownies and disabled Rangers unit gave me the confidence to apply for a Teacher's Training course. Encouraged by friends, I applied to four colleges.

On February 1st 1973 I had an interview at the first college I had chosen. I found it quite easily. It was a new building. I had an appointment with the Vice-principal, Miss Bailey. As I had a disability I needed to seek her approval before meeting the interview panel. Her secretary met me in the carpark. Inside the building, it was difficult to walk because every few yards there were steps without handrails, which affected my balance. I was embarrassed and conscious of my wobbly gait, looking as if I might fall over at any second. I wished this was not so obvious.

'I'm sure Miss Bailey wouldn't mind coming downstairs to see you,' the secretary said several times. 'No, I'm fine.' I tried to sound casual and convincing but I finally gave in and sat down. By repeatedly suggesting I should let Miss Bailey come to me was just reinforcing my severe disability, something I didn't want. Miss Bailey descended the stairs looking thoroughly put out. Somehow I knew this was all a big mistake.

Miss Bailey looked extremely scruffy, considering her important position as Vice-principal. Her hair needed brushing and her clothes were baggy. She looked well past retirement age. She wasn't pleased at having to leave her office to come to see me. I could tell by her expression what she was thinking. I would have no chance of becoming a student in her college if I couldn't even climb stairs to her office. I wanted desperately to train as a teacher. I knew I could cope if given the chance. If only Miss Bailey could see how well children responded to me. Adults have more problems with disabilities than children. I found that children accepted people with a disability in a natural way.

I told Miss Bailey that I was going to see the Assistant Education Officer to discuss my career prospects, and hoped to be allowed to spend some time in a school observing the classes. Miss Bailey said she would like a report from the school. The interview concluded with a promise of another interview with the panel.

Months went by and I waited for my interview. In March, I decided to write to Miss Bailey to find out why I hadn't heard anything. I mentioned I'd spent four full days observing in a local primary school, and recognised that some aspects of teaching might be difficult. Nevertheless, I was confident of overcoming most problems. My letter also described my work with the Brownies and disabled Rangers. I concluded by saying I felt my disabilities looked worse than they really were, which was a great disadvantage. Determined to have an interview with the college panel, I reminded her that I hadn't been notified of the second meeting that she had promised.

My time of observation at the junior school was disappointing. In contrast to the children's friendliness, the staff were distant and cold. In April, two letters arrived: one from the head of the school I had been attending as an observer, and the other from the assistant education officer. They contained the same message. Both said I had the academic ability to teach but seriously doubted whether I could fulfil all the duties expected of a teacher – such as teaching needlework, craft and physical education, or writing comments in children's books or on the blackboard. They also doubted whether I could manage playground duty as I wouldn't be able to separate fighting school children.

The headmaster ended his letter by saying, 'While being sympathetic, in the circumstances I would be reluctant to have you on my staff.'

I shouldn't have been so upset to receive these letters, having already sensed the teachers' attitudes at the school. In contrast support was growing from my college lecturers. My Sociology lecturer telephoned Miss Bailey many times to find out about a date for my interview with the panel without success. She helped me answer letters that raised some valid points. Both the headmaster and education officer had based their findings on assumptions rather than facts. I hadn't been given the opportunity to demonstrate that I could cope with some of the duties listed in the two letters. Craft work and physical exercises were important activities in the Brownie Guide programme.

I wrote to complain that my period of observation at the school had been too brief. I felt that it ought to have been extended to a term, helping as a class assistant. I used my own legible handwriting to prove I was capable of writing comments in children's textbooks.

I am very fortunate that inventiveness often partners the problems brought by disability. I used to help with a Sunday school class. One day as I was walking home from the class I was aware of some children walking behind me. I looked round and was shocked to see they were imitating the way I walked. I was very embarrassed. An idea came to me in a flash. I turned round to face them and spoke. 'Would you children mind walking in front of me please, so that I can try and walk like you?' They instantly walked in front of me. They looked round to see if I was walking like them. It made me smile.

Meanwhile, time was running out. My chances of obtaining a place on a Teacher Training course the following year were fading. I'd applied to three other colleges. My applications obviously hadn't yet been forwarded to them because no decision had been made by my first choice of college. A staff member from Southgate Technical College knew someone in a residential school for girls with disabilities. He arranged for me to spend one day a week assisting in a class for a whole term.

I was encouraged to continue studying for my A levels and apply for a degree course in Humanities. This might give me a better chance to get into teaching. I loved my work in Halliwick School. I worked with two eight-year old girls who had cerebral palsy. Katie and Christine had very little speech. I read to them and discussed the stories, encouraging them to point to words and pictures. Such severely disabled children tend to become withdrawn if left alone without stimulation. These girls came alive in my company, and their faces lit up with excitement. Maybe they were thinking, 'If Joan can work, so too can we, one day.' This was what I really wanted to do – one-to-one teaching with children who badly needed it. I was surprised when their teacher described one girl as having 'a very poor perception of anything other than her immediate surroundings'. Her teacher had to eat her words when this same girl spoke to me from across the classroom one day, and asked in a very clear voice, 'Can we finish that story next week?'

In my final quest to enter the teaching profession, I hoped to get a vote of confidence from a career analyst. I spent a day being interviewed and tested, only to be told in a written report that I had 'unrealistic goals'. He advised me to be satisfied with what I had achieved and to take it easy. He suggested that perhaps I could teach private pupils at home. I'd had a great deal of faith in this man. The Spastics Society had sent me to him and paid for my consultation. I expected him to understand cerebral palsy but the report left me feeling thoroughly demoralised. I felt physically weak and depressed, as if I'd gone down with an attack of 'flu. I felt this way for three weeks. Then it suddenly occurred to me that a brief encounter with one person was not going to change the course of my life. What could he have found out about me in the space of a few hours? Who was an expert in cerebral palsy? What qualifications were required to recognise a person's potential? What greater qualification could there be to help children with disabilities than having lived with cerebral palsy from birth?

And so the fight continued. My Sociology lecturer suggested I take an A level in Sociology to add to my one in English, then apply for a degree course at Middlesex Polytechnic a year later.

19
Middlesex Polytechnic

I chose to apply for the Humanities Degree course at Middlesex Polytechnic in Enfield because it was close to home. I could easily drive there. The advantage of living at home was that I had support from my parents to provide me with care and my meals. I needed to save my energy for my studies.

My interview, in February 1975, took most of the day. The morning was a briefing period for all the students applying for the course. The number of buildings making up the complex was overwhelming. We had to go to different places throughout the day. I had lunch in the refectory. Sitting at the table, I glanced across the room and recognised the familiar face of a student I'd seen earlier on.

He smiled and asked if he could join me. He introduced himself as Philip and said he came from York. Like me, he had found it difficult to find his way around the Poly. We all had interviews that afternoon and were instructed to report to the Tower Block. Philip escorted me to the small seminar rooms. His interview was before mine. At the end of it, he flew out of the room. His face was as white as a sheet, which was scary. He didn't even say goodbye.

The Humanities Degree was made up of modules. I chose English and History as my main subjects. Designing my own degree was very appealing. I chose 17th century poetry, Chaucer's *Canterbury Tales* and plays by Pinter, Miller, Ibsen and Bernard Shaw.

Shakespeare was compulsory. I was told at my interview that they would try and get me double time with a break for my exams. I'd only had 30 minutes extra time when taking my previous exams, which was grossly insufficient. I could type my answers and there was also an option of doing some projects instead of exams. I was allocated my own parking space in a location that was quite central and meant that I could easily reach different buildings. I felt rewarded for all my struggles to obtain the right conditions to minimise the effects of my disability. No more fighting! I could just get on with my studies.

In the few months before my course started, I thought of ways to make life on my course as easy as possible. I needed surgery for carpal tunnel syndrome in my left hand. The NHS kindly obliged and operated a few weeks before I started. Yet I still had my arm in a sling at the start of the induction course. I decided to buy a small shopping trolley to carry my heavy tape recorder and books. The trolley just fitted inside my invalid car and proved to be an invaluable walking aid. Mary, my personal tutor, thought it was an excellent idea. She half-expected other students to follow suit and get themselves trolleys. I found my microphone for recording lectures was too sensitive to being banged on the desk so I attached it to a large sponge with an elastic band.

It was important to learn my way around the campus quickly to save time and energy. I often met students who were lost and helped them find their way around the Poly. I was glad to find that I was among students of a wide age range. Some were much older than I was. What a relief, especially as Mum called me 'the Eternal Student'. It was good to find that Phil was on the same course.

On the Induction Course there were many lectures taking place in large halls at the top of flights of stairs. I waited at the bottom of them with my trolley for some assistance. It was mostly Phil who offered to help. I soon realised that, whenever I was in difficulty, he was always there to help. He would suddenly appear saying in his Irish/Yorkshire accent, 'I'll take that up for you, Joan.'

There were a few visually impaired students on the campus and one other second-year student who'd been badly injured in a car accident. Her obvious struggle to keep up, and flat refusal of help, greatly disturbed both staff and students. One day a tutor said to me in a surprised and somewhat relieved tone, 'You don't mind accepting offers of help do you, Joan?' 'Oh no,' I smiled. 'I need to save my energy as much as possible for my studies.'

All the students in my year looked after me in a kind, un-patronising way. I didn't believe in refusing help in a rude manner. It was hurtful and gave people a bad impression. As people got to know me, they realised I would always ask for help if I needed it. In my second year, Mary, my personal tutor, said that looking after me had brought the students closer together. They always included me in everything.

Tape-recording lectures and seminars meant that all my weekends and evenings were spent making typed notes from tapes. I worked in my bedroom most evenings and Saturdays. My student grant allowed me more money than supplementary benefit, which helped those who couldn't work. I paid for my bedroom to be redecorated in white and yellow to compensate for the lack of sunlight. In addition to my student grant of around £300 a term, I could claim extra money for the petrol I used to travel to my course, and batteries for my tape recorder.

Tape recording lectures took ages. It was a temptation to write every word down. I had never been taught the technique of note taking. My fellow students occasionally asked to borrow my notes by bribing me with a pint of Guinness in the student bar. Only once did I ever have a Guinness but word got around that it was my favourite tipple. I had very little social life. I rarely watched television. In fact, I often had to stop and think what time of year it was – was it nearly Christmas or Easter? At the end of each term there was a disco for my year that I really enjoyed. To my surprise at the first disco Phil sat next to me for the whole evening and subsequently accompanied me to every disco. It was easy to dance to the music of the time: the Beatles, the Rolling Stones, the Beach Boys. Phil always danced with me. I was half-prepared for him to meet another girl and abandon me like Brian had. I was determined to make the most of his friendship. The sad thing was that he was fifteen years younger than I was and I was terrified of him finding out!

Phil was fair and had tight curly hair. What a waste on a boy! He was very shy, but not too shy to wink at me whenever our eyes met. It always made me blush. I liked his sense of humour. Phil could imitate different accents. I always giggled when he talked cockney.

My sister Margaret was now married to Peter who was gentle, kind, and adored Margaret. I wanted to have someone special too. When I told Margaret about Phil, she warned me it wouldn't last. So you can imagine how shocked everyone was when, the following year, he invited me to York for a weekend at his parent's home. Dad said to me before I left, 'Don't let that chap lead you up the garden path.' I travelled there on my own and had a lovely weekend. Phil introduced me to all his friends at the local pub. His Mum and Dad gave me a lovely welcome, his brother and sister too. I'd travelled by train on Friday night. On Saturday, Phil took me out to Castle Howard for a picnic. On Sunday, we walked around the city and had a look at York Minster. We walked along the city wall and along the Shambles looking at the little shops. Phil disappeared into a shop while I waited outside. He returned with a charm for my bracelet, the white rose emblem of Yorkshire. It

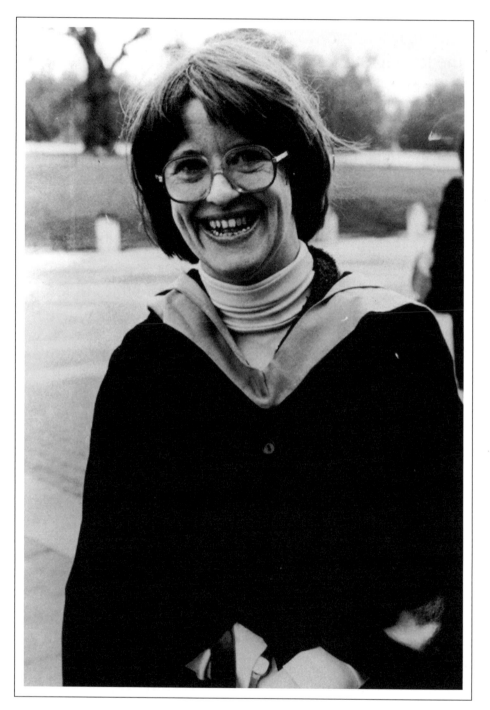

Graduation day, 1978.

made me feel very special. I returned home by train on Sunday, leaving Phil behind as the new term hadn't started yet. This was the first of many annual visits to York, where I always had a wonderful time.

Studying for my degree was very hard work. Nevertheless, it was one of the happiest times of my life. I'd found a place in the able-bodied world.

20
Seeking Employment

During my degree course, I gave up the idea of becoming a teacher. Many friends had become qualified teachers. I received reports of how hard teaching had become, especially with the decline of good behaviour in classrooms.

My tutors at the polytechnic had always told us we were the 'cream of society'. Perhaps they'd falsely given us the impression that prospective employers would welcome us with open arms. I'd gained a 2/2 BA Honours degree in Humanities.

My visit to the Disability Resettlement Officer (DRO) at the job centre soon quashed that illusion. She looked at me despondently, she obviously didn't consider me as employable. I came away with a green card and a number confirming I was registered disabled. I was very disappointed. I later learnt that DROs were more useful after you have found employment. The Department of Employment assisted by providing special equipment if required in the work place, and paid for small adaptations to the building.

I still wanted to work in the disability field and thought about taking a master's degree. It would allow me to research into the needs of children with disabilities coping with integration. It was exciting finding out about the Thomas Coram Institute, attached to London University. In my thesis, I wanted to prove how isolated children were during the weekends and school holidays as special schools and friends were situated far from home. I knew from personal experience how lonely and boring these periods were for them. I was invited to give talks about my childhood to parents of pupils at my old special school. I gathered that parents relied too much on TV to entertain their kids. I wanted to prove the benefit to their children of joining local youth organisations.

At that time, there were no community carers. I was concerned about what might happen to the children if a parent fell ill. Did neighbours know the families well enough, particularly if a disabled child was involved, to assist in an emergency? I was extremely disappointed to find I needed a first class degree to qualify for a grant for further study.

I wrote to the director of Haringey Social Services explaining all about myself. I had never been shown how to write a curriculum vitae. I wrote that I hoped I might be offered a position in the physical disabilities department of Social Services. I was called to an interview with an officer in the department. This two-faced rogue made notes and said he would be in touch if a suitable job came up. It was no surprise that I never heard from him again.

As time went by I wasn't too disappointed that I hadn't yet found work as most of my postgraduate friends, apart from those going on to teacher's training, were also unemployed. I decided to advertise, offering tuition in English language. Two people applied, a boy of thirteen from Mauritius and a young man wanting help with his reading. They were both very nice students. It felt so good to be paid for my skills. I enjoyed preparing the lessons using my English textbooks, even though it took a long time.

The winter months passed. People didn't want to be stuck indoors studying in the summer months. I lost my pupils. I continued to look for employment. It was extremely disappointing to find a lack of advice and support anywhere. It was so different from my days in the polytechnic. I applied for administrative-type jobs, which was probably a mistake. I gained a couple of interviews: one in Environmental Health, a second in a local hospital. By then, it was compulsory to interview a person with a disability.

As the interview for the hospital post progressed, I grew very angry. 'Haven't you read my application form? It doesn't appear so by the type of questions you are asking me.' They looked embarrassed but said nothing. I felt so frustrated I wanted to smash shop windows on my way home. I would have probably failed anyway.

Then my luck changed through a neighbour's kind action. She worked for Islington Council and had a mild disability herself. She spoke to one of the directors on my behalf in Social Services. I was called for an interview and offered a job as a clerical assistant in the Research and Development Department. I was employed through the Special Temporary Employment Programme (STEP), a project that had been set up by the Government, which aimed to place the long-term unemployed in permanent employment.

I was placed in a very friendly office in Islington Park Street. Ken, the Information Officer, supervised me. Lynne, his secretary, also worked for Colin Groves, the Director who had interviewed me. Lorna worked for the Research and Development Officer, and also shared this office.

Ken set me the task of reading newspapers, social work and disability publications, and selecting articles for filing and storing in the library. I photocopied articles of special interest and sent them out to other Social Services departments. This was a familiar task because I had already started a small personal reference library at home, selecting information from the magazines of disability organisations, which I'd joined. I was also allowed to answer the phone and make phone calls.

My work probably developed as a result of the 1970 Chronically Sick and Disabled Person's Act. It transformed the lives of people with an illness or impairment. Local authorities now had a statutory duty to assess their needs, and provide aids and adaptations within the home to assist with daily living. The Government also recognised the financial impact of disability and illness by introducing extra benefits to cover the costs of special diets, heating, laundry, personal care and transport.

When I dropped the phone one day, I feared I'd get fired, as it didn't work so well afterwards. But everyone just laughed, and I was nicknamed 'Wrecker Ross'. Sometimes Ken said with a grin, 'Oh Joan, I wish you hadn't dropped my phone.' Unfortunately I was only allowed to be on the STEP programme for six months. It was such a happy time, working for 35 hours a week at my own pace. Ken once said, 'Joan, if you finish the work in less than the allotted time, you can go home early.' People from other offices popped in to see me, and there were several lunchtime birthday parties.

Towards the end of my six months Ken helped me apply for jobs within the council. He also helped with my curriculum vitae. He found out about another new STEP programme, specifically designed to employ those with a disability to train as advisers to other people with special needs and their carers. It was to be based in Islington under the management of the Greater London Citizen's Advice Bureaux. The work would mainly concentrate on welfare benefits advice over the telephone. At my interview for the job it was both surprising and reassuring to find some people with disabilities on the interview panel.

Melvin Kinnear and I were successful applicants. Our first task was to conduct a feasibility study lasting six months to assess the need for a specialist advice centre on disability benefits. We attended training courses on welfare benefits. Our study demonstrated an overwhelming need for such a centre, so the Advice and Rights Centre for the Handicapped, ARCH, was established, with a further year's funding from a number of large charitable trusts. At last I had the opportunity to work in the disability field after all. It promised to be a fulfilling job.

21
A Real Job

The very first advice centre for people with disabilities and their carers in Islington was to be based at St. John's Day Centre. Some of the users of the centre formed themselves into a Management Committee. Representatives from Islington Disablement Association and the Greater London Association of Citizen's Advice Bureaux were also on the committee.

The Management Committee turned one of the rooms in their day centre into an office for the new advice workers. It was a large, roomy office with a long worktop along the length of one wall. Melvin and I kept our typewriter and files there. There was enough space on the worktop for us to make tea and coffee. We sat facing one another at our large desks. We each had a telephone. One management committee member, who was an artist, designed a logo for ARCH. The logo was a telephone with 'ARCH' printed on its dial.

One of our first visitors was the Disablement Resettlement Officer (DRO). Melvin was a wheelchair user, paralysed from the neck down. The DRO suggested we both had special hands free telephones, which enabled us to make notes while on the telephone. We had a kettle tipper to assist pouring boiling water to make our drinks. We were granted electric typewriters because of our writing difficulties. In due course the gadgets arrived. The special telephone was excellent. The receiver was replaced by a weight on the phone. It was clamped onto a stand that could be moved near the ear.

Melvin and I were asked to spend the first six months conducting a feasibility study proving the need for the service. We also had to attend training courses on welfare rights provided by the Citizens Advice Bureau (CAB). We were visited regularly by one of the workers from the local CAB who supervised our work.

We had to create an information resource for our enquirers. We visited a few organisations for disability, including the Royal Association for Disability and Rehabilitation (RADAR). We had a visit from a member of the Disability Advice Line (DIAL). Individual people started DIAL, working voluntarily from their own homes, giving advice and information to people with disabilities. It grew into a national organisation called DIAL UK. We were both increasingly convinced of the need for an advice and information service.

Six months later we opened up to the public. It was important to keep records of our calls. The statistics could be used for getting more funding after the STEP government funding ended. Often, calls were not directly about benefits. Sometimes a caller had a phone bill or gas bill they couldn't afford to pay. Further questions revealed the caller wasn't claiming all the benefits they were entitled to. A leaflet was sent to them explaining benefit entitlement. Sometimes a letter was written to the Social Security office on their behalf. I always feared being asked a question I couldn't answer. At our training courses we were told to deal with this by saying to the enquirer, 'I don't know but I will find out for you and phone you back.' Melvin and I relied on the Disability Rights Handbook, which had first been produced by The Disability Alliance in 1978. We called this useful handbook, which was updated every year in line with the changes in the benefit system, our 'Bible'. The number of telephone enquiries grew steadily. We received calls from people living outside the borough. We trained volunteers from St. John's Day Centre to help in the office.

Melvin and I, despite our age difference, worked well together. Melvin picked up the benefit system very quickly and I often felt undermined by his superior knowledge. It was a very new subject to me. Melvin, aged about 23, had been paralysed through a diving accident. He was one of the few people I met who was newly disabled. Most of my friends were disabled from birth. I learnt a lot about problems people faced being newly disabled. Melvin had spent a long time in Stoke Mandeville Hospital, and was now living in a hostel for physically disabled people. He came to work every day by minicab and was financially assisted by the Department of Employment's 'Fares to Work Scheme'.

Melvin was about six-foot tall, he had big, brown eyes and very dark, curly hair that he wore at shoulder length. Once I felt very let down by Melvin when one morning he called me at work. 'Joan I'm not coming to work today,' he said, 'I'm supporting the public workers' strike.' I was extremely shocked and angry. I managed to ask, 'Will you be in tomorrow then?' He said he would. I carried on with my usual work. I knew it was wrong of him to strike.

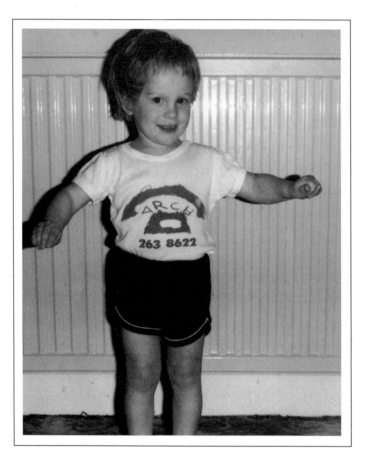

My nephew Andrew in his ARCH
tee-shirt, 1980.

We didn't even belong to a union. We were on a special government scheme and weren't being paid by the council.

The next morning, Melvin turned up for work. How could I show him how angry I was? I decided not to speak to him. I don't really sulk but it was the only weapon I could think of. It created a very dark atmosphere, which even felt eerie to me! Melvin slowly and quietly moved around the office in his wheelchair with his head slightly bent. I thought he made a very good impersonation of someone tiptoeing around the room feeling guilty. Then he asked, 'Are you all right, Joan?' A whole torrent of abuse poured out of my mouth, which I can't possibly repeat. Melvin said defensively, 'I was in the pub the night before last with a few friends. Everyone was talking about the strike and how important it was to take action. I really felt that I should go on strike too.' 'But, Melvin, neither of us are in a union,' I said. 'Also, we're trying desperately to create a valuable advice and information centre. It's important that we prove ourselves as good employees.'

Sadly our year came to an end as no further funding materialized, despite complete recognition of our success. We were unemployed once again. We didn't want to see ARCH close down, so Melvin and I offered to continue working as volunteers. One social services area team put both of us on their volunteer list, and paid us £5 a week as volunteers for ARCH. This at least covered my petrol costs. We both claimed unemployment benefit again. This time, I signed on by post for my benefit. I refused to do this at the beginning. I went to sign on every fortnight. I thought that if I were unable to get to the office to sign on, people would think that I couldn't get to my work place.

While Melvin and I continued to work voluntarily for ARCH, the management committee continued to find another organisation to fund us with the help of Greater London Organisation of Citizen's Advice Bureaux (GLOCABS). In 1981 we were approaching the first International Year of Disabled People. I.Y.D.P. was a major step in putting disability issues on the agenda. There were many documentaries about disability on television. A number of disabled people were interviewed. At last disability was being given a high profile.

I encouraged the management committee to fundraise for ARCH. We had a raffle and I donated Easter eggs as prizes. No one ever thought of registering ARCH as a charity. A friend managed to get a benefit concert put on for ARCH in her local church, which was very successful at raising money. Some of its success was due to a husband and wife team of opera singers from the Royal Opera House, Covent Garden. We also sold t-shirts, sweat shirts and badges displaying the ARCH logo.

At around the same time the Greater London Council (GLC) started funding voluntary organisations. The ARCH Management committee put in an application for funding to resume having paid workers. It took several months for news of funding to come through.

I was amazed at the differences in provision of services for disabled people in Islington compared with Haringey where I lived. As indicated, there was already a thriving disability association in Islington. Islington had a Dial-A-Ride service. There was also 'Crossroads' providing relief for carers in their own home. The hostel where Melvin lived was another impressive establishment for people with disabilities, enabling them to have control of their own care as far as possible. I was most impressed with the work carried out in St. John's Day Centre for people with special needs. There were none of these services in Haringey.

After 1981 Haringey was at last catching up in provision. An Occupational Therapist from Haringey came to see me in ARCH to find out about its work. There were rumblings of a disability association being started. Soon there was news of a telephone help-line to be manned by volunteers with a disability. Haringey Social Services set up meetings with people with disabilities to plan starting up a disabilities association. First, a Handicapped Information Telephone Service was created. Then, surprise, surprise, I was headhunted for the post of Advice Officer for Haringey Disabilities Association. I had to make a difficult decision on whether to stay with ARCH, and see if the GLC followed through with funding for Melvin and me to become full-time workers again. I couldn't really take that chance so I accepted the post of Advice Officer in Haringey. I had a real job at last, working for17.5 hours a week. After I had left, the GLC did eventually provide funding for ARCH. Melvin continued to work there.

In 1979, something wonderful happened. My sister presented me with a nephew named Andrew. It was lovely to earn enough money and make regular visits to Mothercare to buy him Babygros in a variety of colours. Three years later, I also had a niece named Gemma.

22
Haringey Disability Association

I was surprised to see John Hall on the interview panel for my new job. He was one of the residential children on the Cerebral Palsy Unit in Queen Mary's Hospital, Carshalton. It's a small world! I had met with John and his wife Yvonne at some of the meetings in Haringey during International Year of Disabled People. During the interview, John asked me the toughest questions, spelling them out on his alphabet board because of his speech problems.

I started work in September 1982. The Haringey Disability Association was given offices in a hut at the back of Tottenham Town Hall. It consisted of a large room with several offices leading off. It was the same building where I had had an interview with an officer from Social Services soon after graduating. The building was cold in winter, often the central heating wasn't working properly. In summer wasps liked to nest in the roof and often plagued us.

I was job-sharing with Anne Gardner who wasn't disabled. We worked 17.5 hours a week. We had a manager, Jane McVeigh. Lynne Davies, the

Administration Assistant, also had a disability. The fourth member of staff, Liz Worsley, was the Community Development Officer. We were all new members of staff in a new organisation.

At first I found it quite stressful working alongside an able-bodied person. I felt very aware of how quick and dextrous Anne was. She could do several tasks at once with great speed. I felt threatened by her capabilities until I realised that what I lacked physically was compensated by my knowledge of disability and its issues.

A year later after HDA opened we had another administration person joining the team. Rena looked after the Management Committee and collected membership fees. Rena was a very jolly person, welcoming everyone who called at the office. She looked after me supplying me with cups of tea and coffee throughout the day. Sharing the drink making facilities with other people made it difficult for me to make my own drinks because I needed to have everything set out in a certain way and to use a kettle tipper.

It was good to have a manager to supervise my work. It brought more professionalism into it. For the first six months Anne and I worked together on the same days. During this time we planned the nature of our work and visited voluntary and statutory organisations in the borough, telling them about our work. Six months later we officially opened the advice service and worked on separate days. On Wednesdays we worked together taking the opportunity to inform each other about work matters. This was also the day when we held our staff meetings.

The Handicapped Information Telephone Service volunteers came to join us in the afternoons. Two volunteers came in to oversee the service. The office that I worked in was very small. It was very cramped sharing with two volunteers. I'm sure the volunteers did a very good job giving advice and help over the telephone. As we were now part of a large organisation, the kind of enquiries became more complex and needed more specialist help. For example, there was an elderly lady looking after her son with a disability and her husband had become incontinent after a stroke. She had to go to the laundrette every day. I contacted the social services and managed to get her a washing machine.

We ran training courses for the volunteers, improving their approach to the advice work. I have to say that these conditions were not ideal for advice work. It was a great relief when the telephone service was disbanded, leaving the advice work to Anne and me. We still used volunteers to do some typing and general office work

HDA had a Management Committee elected from its membership made up of individuals and groups representing people with disabilities. Pam Moffatt became the first Chairperson. Pam was a force to be reckoned with. Although a Haringey resident, she had worked for many years in Islington Disablement Association. At last people living in Haringey would benefit from Pam's energetic driving force to obtain services for people with special needs. Although severely disabled herself, Pam spoke so commandingly, no one dared disagree with her.

HDA's Management Committee's first task was to find funds to set up a Dial-a-Ride and a Care Attendant Scheme in Haringey (a scheme to help carers). Haringey Council only provided funding for the salaries of the core staff including myself.

I was asked to represent HDA on the councils' Social Services Committee as a co-opted member from a voluntary organisation. This was very interesting work. A few days before the committee meeting I received the committee papers. Jane McVeigh went over the papers with me. Each committee report had a comment about how it effected ethnic minority groups and other groups. There was no mention of disability as part of these comments. It was my task to remind the committee to put a comment about disability at the end of these reports. At every meeting I reminded the committee to include special needs in the reports. Eventually they took this on board and included it on their papers. Disability issues surfaced quite often at the committee meetings: home care, day centres and plans for residential care and sheltered housing schemes. I often thought of questions relating to these projects that had been overlooked in some areas.

Within a couple of years the HDA had found agencies to fund Dial-a-Ride and a Care Attendant Scheme. Haringey Council provided funding to employ two

144

workers with disabilities as Access Officers to improve access to public buildings.

The HDA produced its own monthly magazine for its membership. I often wrote articles giving information on disability issues and benefits. After about three years we had a new manager, Colin Anderson. He arrived at the same time as computers, which were becoming an essential part of office equipment. It was like a revolution. Colin knew a lot about computers and we all went on training courses to learn more about them. I had to wait a long time before the Employment Service replaced my electric typewriter with my own computer. It greatly improved the quality of my work. The computer meant that we could produce a much smarter magazine for our members. The front cover was now glossy, and often had a photograph. This was largely due to Colin's computer skills. I really felt proud of our magazine that represented a highly professional organisation supporting people with disabilities.

Anne Gardener left us after two years and Dennis Goldstein replaced her as Advice Officer. Dennis had a hidden disability. This American gentleman possibly in his forties was quiet and gentle. He had been a social worker and had an oblique sense of humour! He came to work by public transport, quite a journey from West Hampstead. He kept himself going by drinking endless cups of coffee but was reluctant to make me a cup, which was quite hurtful, especially as I couldn't make it myself.

As more people came into the office for advice, preferring not to use the telephone, we started using an appointment system and developing casework. Once we started working with somebody we kept records about our clients and people had their individual preferences about which advice officer they wanted to help them. This system worked quite well.

23
Changing Cars

While I was working voluntarily for ARCH I decided it was time to think about driving a four-wheel car instead of my invalid car. I had been driving a long time now. It was a disadvantage not to take passengers in the invalid car. Also, they were quite dangerous to drive in bad weather.

It was quite a gamble to make this change. I would have to take the full driving test and in order to afford a new adapted car I would have to exchange my invalid car for the mobility allowance. I had to decide whether it was worth taking the risk of forfeiting my invalid car for the mobility allowance. There was no guarantee that I would be able to drive an ordinary car even with the adaptations. The charity Motability was set up by the Government to assist people with disabilities who qualify for the mobility allowance. There was a six-month period allowing me to keep my invalid car and claim mobility allowance. This would help me to make up my mind about driving another car.

First I applied to Motability and enrolled with British School of Motoring (BSM) who boasted that they could teach anyone with a disability to drive. They had specially adapted cars for the purpose of learning. I found a local BSM instructor and arranged a lesson. Foolishly, I paid him for a month's lessons as a sign of my commitment to learn to drive and looked forward to my first lesson.

On that first lesson I sat in the driving seat learning to use the controls. It was an automatic car. It had left foot controls and a knob on the steering wheel. Most drivers with a disability needed hand controls. I was very fortunate that I was able to learn on a car with these left foot controls. I wasn't so fortunate with the instructor. He seemed a bundle of nerves. I wonder why! He was a chain smoker. On my second lesson I actually drove the car. It was a hair-raising experience! The instructor remained very quiet. I felt very uneasy, I realised I was driving badly. When I recognised I'd done something well I craved for a crumb of encouragement from him but he remained silent. 'I did that well didn't I?' I bleated hopefully but only got a, 'Hmmm,' by reply. I was determined not to give up just yet. Towards the end of the first month my instructor was keen to remind me it was time to pay for more lessons. If only he had put the same enthusiasm into teaching me to drive as he did into getting more money out of me.

Motability eventually arranged for me to have an assessment on my driving and the kind of adaptations needed for my car. BSM had a special assessment centre in Wimbledon for this purpose. I arranged for a friend to come with me for this assessment to provide me with transport. There was heavy traffic on the way to Wimbledon. On arrival I could have done with a cup of coffee to set me up for this ordeal. No such luck! A tall man came over and in a patronising voice said, 'Will you accompany me to the car park, dear?' I was led like a lamb to the slaughter to a large car and told to sit in the driver's seat. 'Will you start the car, dear? Check your mirrors and follow my directions.' Before I knew it I found myself driving up Wimbledon High Street in a stream of traffic approaching a large roundabout where I managed to stop and wait for a clear entry. Suddenly my foot jerked and I pressed the accelerator and shot forward in the car. The instructor responded by braking using the dual controls. He drove me back to the centre. I felt like a very naughty child. There was no discussion about what happened. I felt terrible and a complete failure.

Back at home when things had calmed down a little and I reflected on what happened, I felt the whole assessment had been very badly planned and unfair to me. I should have been told exactly what was going to be required of me so that I could assess my own capability to carry it out. When I reported the incident to my instructor his manner toward me was more depressing than ever. I decided this person wasn't going to succeed in teaching me to drive. I called it a day and stopped the driving lessons. I decided to save up for my own car, have it adapted, and find myself a kind and understanding instructor.

Two years later I had enough money to put a deposit on a new Mini Mayfair on a hire purchase scheme. I paid for the adaptations. It had an automatic transmission.

I needed the pedals changed so that I could use them with my left foot. I also had a steering wheel knob put on. This work was done in a specialist garage near Hanger Lane. Fortunately I still had my invalid car, because I didn't go into the Motability Scheme. There was a small driving school in my area called Bryan J's. They advertised driving lessons for people with a disability. The school had a special car with hand controls.

I arranged to have lessons from Bryan J's using my own car. Andy, my instructor, was so different from the first one I had. This friendly middle-aged man from Greece immediately put me at my ease. I felt relaxed with him. He was obviously very committed to teaching people with disabilities. He said I was a challenge to him. He wouldn't have found it easy to teach me to drive had I not driven already. I had gained road sense and an understanding of how other drivers behave. This left me free to concentrate on gaining full control of the car. It was much harder than driving the invalid car. I had to learn to touch the pedals very lightly because the car was so powerful and would shoot forward with very little pressure. Once more, at home, I got my big sponge out and practised pressing my foot lightly just as I would on the pedal.

I chose a Mini because I thought it would be easy to steer. This was a mistake. A small car requires many more turns of the steering wheel. The hardest thing was to make right hand turns. I found it very hard to turn the wheel round far enough. Because of this I failed my first driving test. The examiner recommended installing power steering. This would be very expensive. Andy recognised my difficulty. His solution was to place the steering wheel knob further back on the wheel to help me turn it more easily. It was then much easier to turn the steering wheel.

While I was learning to drive I was fortunate enough to be able to drive to and from work every day. My work was situated five miles from home. Dad had now retired and kindly accompanied me to and from work each day. He returned home by bus and came back for me in the evening. Driving every day with Dad as well as having a weekly driving lesson was good experience for me. I think Dad was very proud of me. I used to hear him telling other people that I worked and drove on one of the busiest roads in North London.

Six months later I took my driving test again and passed. It was wonderful, one of the best things that had happened to me in my life! I could now go on holiday in my own car with Janet. I discovered that it was possible to put the car on the motor rail and go all the way to Scotland. We had quite a few lovely holidays there.

I was very proud of my little car. It was dark blue and I was able to help Dad wash and polish it. Best of all it had a radio and a tape recorder. I found it very relaxing to listen to my favourite music. It seemed to keep me calm and drowned out any sudden noises from other vehicles.

Mum was beginning to get arthritis in her knees and I was able to take her around in my car. The journey to my sister's was quite busy. I didn't like Dad driving us. I managed to persuade my parents to let me drive them on our visit to our family in Walthamstow. I could see my Dad in my rear view mirror looking rather miserable in the back seat. He really didn't like being driven.

I loved driving and felt very rewarded for my hard work towards learning to drive. However, one day I had a very bad accident on my way to work, only a few yards from home. Suddenly my car went out of control and I went off the road, across the pavement and onto a service road. I just managed to stop against the wall of the pub. In the crash I had smashed my headlights. The landlady from the pub came out to see what had happened. There was no damage to the pub wall. An old man passed shaking his head saying, 'You should call the police.' The landlady dismissed this idea. She took me inside and made me a cup of coffee. She was so understanding. I thought I must have hit the accelerator pedal by mistake. She said that a similar thing had happened to her. In fact, the right foot pedal was held out of the way by a clip and the clip had broken. It came down giving me two accelerator pedals! The car had been adapted in this way to enable someone else to drive the car. I had the spare pedal removed.

I felt better and continued my journey to work feeling very sad and ashamed by the accident. My manager, Colin, cheered me up when he said, 'I've heard of people calling into the pub on their way home from work. I have never known anyone to call in the pub on their way to work, Joan!'

When I took the car to the garage to get an estimate for the damage there were a few mechanics working on cars outside. They knew me and stopped working to watch me drive my poor car in. It was so embarrassing.

24
My Small Corner

The management committee wanted to develop the organisation further by making it into an umbrella organisation for all other groups representing disability in the borough. The membership was open to groups and individuals. These were represented on our management committee. Soon there were plans to have a purpose built building for HDA. The association also changed its name to Haringey Disabilities Consortium (HDC). A new building was indeed very exciting news. A few sites in the borough were identified for this purpose and a building fund was set up.

Eventually a suitable building to house all our staff was found in the late 1980s. Situated in Bruce Grove on Tottenham High Road it was in a shopping area easily accessible to the public. It once belonged to the Water Board. We moved in 1990. Most of the building was open plan. Dennis Goldstein and I were fortunate to have our own office on the front of the building. It was light and airy with large windows, a pleasant change compared with our small office in Tottenham Town Hall. The office met all the needs of our work. It was soundproof, which was essential to the highly confidential and sensitive work we were now undertaking. When I was a little girl, you will remember my mention of my 'small corner' in the living room where I kept and played with my toys. This was now my new 'small corner'. This is where God had placed me. My disappointments and achievements put me in a good position to give others courage and confidence to overcome their difficulties and achieve their goals.

My main work was to assist people in applying for the two main disability benefits: Attendance Allowance for people needing help with personal care and/or supervision and Mobility Allowance for people who are virtually unable to walk or need supervision out of doors for their own safety. When these benefits were first introduced the application form consisted of just two pages requiring very little information about the person. A retired doctor was often employed to visit them at home. The claimant usually found the visit quite an ordeal. The doctor asked very few questions and made a few notes in a scrawl difficult to read which had to be signed by the claimant. Many claimants were turned down for the benefit.

At this stage these people contacted us for advice. People complained to me that the doctor had not appeared to be listening to anything that was said to him or her. When they received a letter giving reasons for being turned down for the benefit, the person realised that the statement they had signed said that they could walk at least 100 yards without pain or discomfort. The problem was that the claimant probably found it difficult to read the doctor's statement before signing and felt too embarrassed to say so.

Dennis and I were able to help people appeal by asking them to describe a typical walk, and to include the distance and at what stage they became tired and any pain started or got worse. This information had to be as accurate as possible. To support this information we would try and obtain medical evidence from the person's doctor or hospital consultant. We used the same method for appealing against a refusal for the Attendance Allowance. For this we often asked people to keep diaries. This was particularly useful for people whose condition varied from day to day and for those whose need for attention varied from night to night. The diary was particularly valuable for parents of children with special needs. With this kind of information the Department of Health and Social Security called the applicant to attend an appeals tribunal. It was quite a challenge representing people at an appeals tribunal. I could only do this if I had sufficient medical evidence and/or good diaries to support the appeal. I'm pleased to say I had a very good success rate. When I first attended the tribunals I appeared to have more mobility problems than the person I was representing and on some occasions the tribunal clerk asked me if I was claiming the Mobility Allowance!

In due course, these two benefits (the Attendance Allowance and Mobility Allowance) had a new name called the Disability Living Allowance. A new form was introduced, about 36 pages long, to claim both benefits.

Depending on the severity of the disability it could take up to four hours to complete. I thought that this form was excellent because it allowed people to present a complete picture of their condition. However, when it was realised how many questions there were to answer, people got very tired of going through it. It usually had to be done over a period of three to four separate appointments. Very often I was helping people whose English was their second language. I had to dictate the answers for them, often spelling out most of the words. In this situation filling in the application form took even longer. I also liked to photocopy these forms for future reference in case we needed to go to a tribunal. I found it very worth while assisting people apply for DLA. I had a few people with very complex impairments and care problems. I often had to devise unusual methods to prove their needs by seeking further evidence from other professional people involved with the person. Another new benefit introduced around the same time also needed these same methods of proof. It was called Incapacity Benefit, requiring proof for people who were unfit to work. Quite a few people suffering from Myalgic Encephalomyelitis (ME) approached me. This was another illness that wasn't accepted as genuine in the 1980s. However my experience proved successful in gaining benefit for ME sufferers too.

Sadly, in the early 1990s, Dennis died suddenly from a massive heart attack. The Haringey Disabilities Consortium (HDC) decided not to replace Dennis but to create a new post with that money, so I became the only Advice Officer. We also had a new manager, Margaret

Riley. Margaret insisted on very detailed statistics from the advice service for funding purposes, expanding my work further. Regretfully the extra paperwork gave me less time for the advice work.

When people visited me they didn't expect to be helped by a person with a severe disability. Often I recognised how pleased they were to talk to someone who understood their problems. Some people wanted to be able to get their own car through Motability and learn to drive. They needed reassuring that this could be done. I was able to tell them how I had gone through the process of learning to drive, giving them the relevant information. People also wanted to know where they could go on holiday including suitable accommodation. Often I was able to recommend places I had stayed myself.

I suspected that a small minority of people wanted to exaggerate their disability in order to claim the increased number of benefits available to them. This may have been due to a lack of opportunities in employment for people with special needs, or the low basic rate of income support. A young girl came to my office wanting to claim Mobility Allowance because she had a back injury from a car accident. During our interview I was amazed to find the amount of painkillers she was taking, which was resulting in her sleeping most of the day. 'You are taking far too many painkillers, it's no wonder you spend most of your life sleeping,' I told her in a concerned tone. 'Do you really need to take all these tablets?' I said, suggesting that she might look into an alternative way of controlling pain. I wrote to her hospital consultant. I wasn't surprised that he didn't support her claim for Mobility Allowance. A few months later when I arrived at work one morning, I recognised a pretty young girl smiling at me, sitting behind a computer. It was the same young lady. She had come to work with us for the day as an office temp. I was delighted that this young lady had taken a leaf out of my book and was now working just like me in my 'small corner.'

25
Concern Over My Parents' Health

When Mum turned 70 there was a noticeable change in her health. This healthy woman who had never gone to the doctor, except when she was pregnant with Margaret, suddenly became pale and lethargic. There was a noticeable loss of weight. It was suspected that she might have diabetes but all the tests proved negative until a sore appeared on her foot. A further test proved positive: she had diabetes. Within a few days however, she looked a lot better after taking insulin in tablet form.

Dad, now aged 74, caught shingles which left him with eczema. Afterwards, there was a permanent decline in his health. Mum started complaining of pain in her hip and was referred to a surgeon for a hip replacement. Mum and Dad had been on a few holidays by coach in Spain. They thought this was the easiest way to travel for Mum because there was less walking involved. When Margaret and I were young Dad took us by car all over the continent as far as Yugoslavia. We had some lovely holidays.

The year that Dad had shingles he cancelled his holiday to Spain on the very day they should have left. It showed how unwell he was to have cancelled it, even though he had recovered from shingles some time ago. He always loved his holidays and looked forward to them so much. Mum continued to complain about the pain in her hip. It seemed to change her whole personality. She became very demanding towards Dad. She sent him out shopping, got him to pay the rent and collect the weekly pension. At first he managed very well. Physically he was able to walk very fast and appeared to be quite fit. When he became a little forgetful he wrote shopping lists and other notes to remind him of things that he had to do.

I took on responsibility for the main shopping and had most of it delivered. Mum no longer got up to make my breakfast before I went to work, Dad made it. I helped him sort out the medication for himself and my mother after breakfast every day. It was very unfortunate that Mum had diabetes because she had a very sweet tooth and loved fresh cream and jam sponges. Dad was very strict with Mum about keeping to her sugar-free diet to keep her diabetes under control.

We were all very concerned with the increasing pain in Mum's hip. She screamed and winced with pain. Several hospital admissions for a hip replacement were cancelled. She'd been waiting nearly two years. Dad, in his quiet way, kept his concerns to himself. One day he went off somewhere for a few hours. Nobody knew where he had gone. When he came back he announced he'd been all the way to the Royal Free Hospital in Hampstead insisting on seeing Mum's consultant, unannounced of course. A few days later a letter came with a date for Mum's admission for the operation. I was amazed that Dad had managed to get her admitted so quickly. Being a reticent man he never told us what he'd said to her consultant but it certainly did the trick.

The operation was a great success. All the pain in Mum's hip seemed to cease. During her recovery period I arranged for a care attendant to come and cook some meals for us all during the week. Two ladies came on separate days and cooked a roast Sunday lunch, egg and chips on Mondays and another roast dinner on Wednesdays. It was very valuable to me to come home to a cooked meal on two out of the three days I worked. On the other days we managed between us to cook a simple meal every day. Mum and Dad didn't really take to the idea of having other people coming into the home to help them but the two ladies who came to help were extremely nice and Mum and Dad grew to like and accept them quickly. It helped that I ensured that they cooked the meals exactly the same way as Mum did. We were very lucky to have this help.

We didn't keep the care attendants for very long because Mum's hip replacement was so successful. Within a year however, Mum started complaining about her knee being very painful to the extent that, once more, her mobility was seriously affected. She had her second operation quite quickly. The operation was scheduled for a Wednesday. We were horrified to hear it was cancelled at the eleventh hour, after she had been given her pre-med! No explanation was given. She was operated on two days later by a different surgeon again with no explanation as to why this had happened. Dad visited her on his own on the Saturday. He was very quiet after returning home. I didn't really give this much thought. My sister, her family and I all visited Mum on the Sunday afternoon expecting to see her sitting up in bed, her usual cheerful self. Instead, we were shocked to find her in a cot and delirious. Her knee was attached to a machine to exercise it. She was struggling to get her leg free from it and was very distressed. It was awful to see her in such a confused state. Being a Sunday only a few young nurses were on duty on the ward. There was no one qualified to explain the reason for my mother's distressing condition. It was a terrible shock for us all. I burst into tears to see my poor Mum like this. She was always so bright and alert. I was worried about my niece and nephew, Andrew and Gemma, seeing their poor Granny in this situation. They were still very young. All we could do was return home and suffer a sleepless night, waiting until Monday morning to find out what was wrong. Margaret was told that the operation and drugs had upset my Mother's sugar level and caused the delirium. Concern over her diabetes was possibly why the first surgeon had cancelled her operation. It took around ten days for Mum to recover back to her usual self although, sadly, she had deteriorated mentally.

Back at home, the knee operation wasn't quite as successful as the hip operation had been. Mum could no longer do the cooking and cleaning. The care attendants returned to give us their valuable help. We had a new Italian helper, named Italia. She was an angel. Mum soon accepted her and thought she was wonderful. She treated our home as her own, keeping it clean and tidy, doing things in excess of what was required of her. Italia had a daughter with profound disabilities who had recently passed away in her early 20s. She'd provided her with total care. To aid her recovery from this sad loss Italia had started helping families care for their relative with a disability. Italia is still my carer today. Needless to say, she is an excellent carer because she really has her heart in what she does.

There followed nearly five years of heartache and stress, witnessing a gradual loss of mental and physical function in both my parents. This is when mourning begins and death is just a happy release. There was the slow realisation that I had to care for Mum and Dad. Returning the care they'd given me was of course a privilege. Nevertheless, feeling physically and financially independent, part of me longed to set myself up in a home of my own in a place where I could entertain my friends, explore my creativity and find someone to share my life with. Someone as lovely as Phil but nearer to my own age.

I was amazed and very proud of what I was able to do for my parents. My sister did what she could. Living some distance away and having two young children made it difficult. Living with my parents meant I had to 'face the music' alone. I was determined not to give up work.

26
Problems at Home

When Dad retired, I became the centre of his life. I was glad of his help: taking me out to my car, opening the garage doors for me and carrying my bags. The whole street must have known when I was taking my car out of the garage, as Dad shouted, 'Turn the wheel more to the right. Woah! Stop!' He totally confused me. When he saw me turn on my car radio and wave goodbye, he frowned with disapproval. He didn't think I should be listening to the radio as it might distract me from driving.

He started to wait for me to come home so that he could help me in, and I felt under pressure to be home on time. If I were late, he became distressed. I would occasionally go out for meals with graduate friends. Dad's idea of going out for a meal was to go out, eat your meal, pay for it and return straight home again. He imagined I'd be home within an hour. It was all very worrying. The only thing I could do was to add two or three hours to the time I told him I would return home. I was very concerned in winter when I arrived home to find him standing outside in the cold. Things became worse when Dad lost account of time. The carers told me that he insisted on going outside to wait for me at 5 p.m. I didn't leave work till 5.30 p.m. and never reached home until 6 p.m.

Dad started to lose his keys and his bus pass. Sometimes, he was fortunate and had the bus pass posted back to him by an honest person. He grew tired of having to go back and get a new bus pass every time he lost one, so he walked everywhere. To overcome the problem of losing his flat keys he tied them to his belt. This helped, until he got tired of doing it. Instead, he wedged the doors with some paper every time he went out, which the neighbours didn't appreciate as our block of flats had an intercom entry system.

One day, when I was going out to do some shopping, Dad as usual came with me to help get my car out of the garage. As we left, two smartly dressed men walked briskly towards us and made for the door we'd just come through. I turned round and watched them suspiciously.

Then I shouted, 'Dad, get back indoors! I think those men have gone into our flat.' I went shopping, confident Dad had seen these two men off the premises. When I returned home an hour later, Mum said a very nice man had come to mend our dripping tap in the kitchen. Looking round the flat I found my dressing-table drawer open and missing money. My dressmaking case, which was very hard to open, had a hole in the lid and a bread knife beside it. The case was heavy as it contained a sewing tin full of cotton reels, scissors, and buttons. They must have thought it had contained jewellery or money.

168

The loss of money, and the fact that two con men had entered our flat, was nothing compared to the startling realisation that Mum and Dad had no conception of what had happened. I spent the whole weekend trying to make Mum understand but she wouldn't believe me.

'You know the kitchen tap has been dripping for ages,' Mum said, 'and I've been waiting for somebody to come and mend it.'

Not true. Dad didn't say anything about the two men. Had Mum and Dad deteriorated mentally as well as physically? I hadn't realised that the problem was so serious. I'd need help to look after them. Community care provision from the council had not yet been introduced. I was terribly worried about going to work and leaving them alone all day. My sister lived too far away to pop in, and she was tied up with taking the children to and from school every day.

Somehow I had to stop Dad coming out with me to help me. I devised ways of diverting his attention to something else, whilst I slipped out of the front door to go to work. My favourite ploy was to ask him to water the window boxes for me on the two balconies. This worked for a while until Mum realised he wasn't helping me and sent him after me. When I saw him coming I panicked and shouted at him to go back indoors. The poor man got so upset with Mum telling him one thing and me another. I really needed his support and he was very cross that I rejected his help.

Ideally I needed a carer to be at home with my parents during the daytime, or perhaps they could go to a day-centre. Fortunately there was a centre run by Age Concern very near to where we lived. I managed to persuade Mum and Dad to go to it for one afternoon a week but Dad left and came home again. I didn't want him to be home on his own. I asked Italia to come and help my mum get ready. One of the centre helpers called to take her. Italia stayed with Dad. This was only a partial solution to the pressing problem of their daily care.

It was strange coming in from work in the evening. I longed to know what had happened during the day. Had any one called? Were there any telephone messages? No one could tell me. How I missed the chats with Mum over a cup of tea at bedtime. There was just silence now except for the television. Mum and Dad sat in front of it, looking so frail. Mum insisting on having the gas fire on even in summer.

It was suggested that I apply for a grant to employ a carer from the Independent Living Fund. In fact Mum was the only eligible person to apply for this grant. I had to see a social worker to help me make the application, which would include a care plan for my Mother. It took a whole year for this application to go through. I also applied for the attendance allowance for both parents. It was embarrassing when the visiting doctors came to assess my parents. They seemed so normal.

Mum said to the doctor and her GP on several occasions, 'We're alright! It's her that needs help,' pointing at me. 'We look after her!'

I wasn't sure whether or not the doctors believed her, as she spoke with such conviction. Thankfully, we did get the middle rate attendance allowance for both parents. When the ILF money came through, it only allowed enough money to cover seven hours' paid help but this was better than nothing. I had to concentrate all the hours into the period when I worked. I was imprisoned in my home looking after my parents from Thursday until Monday when I returned to work. I used the attendance allowance money for some extra hours of care to cover some gaps in the hours I was at work. When I was stuck at home with my parents I found it too stressful to be in the same room with them all the time. I stayed in the kitchen and listened to books on tape, which helped to pass the time.

Dad came into the kitchen from time to time. I asked, 'What do you want Dad?' I knew what was coming, which was another reason for my being in the kitchen. 'Your Mother wants me to peel some potatoes for dinner,' he said. 'Look, Dad, you've already done them.' I pointed to a saucepan full of peeled potatoes on the gas stove. One day, I had found three saucepans full of peeled potatoes, ready for dinner.

I wished I had the magic drink Alice had in Alice in Wonderland, to make me small enough to sit on Dad's shoulder all day, giving him instructions and advice to keep him safe.

Mum's diabetes made her feet very sore and uncomfortable, although there was nothing to see. The doctor prescribed some cream to soothe them. She would ask Dad to put some cream on her feet several times a day. One day, to my horror, I caught Dad putting toothpaste on her feet instead of cream! He'd obviously had difficulty finding the cream and had thought toothpaste would do instead. Poor Dad; I had to hide the toothpaste in case it caused more irritation on Mum's sore feet.

I was proud and amazed that I was able to look after my parents. Even though it was frightening at times, I didn't resent any of it. They had done so much for me.

27
Voluntary Work

Between 1963 and 1975 I was Assistant Guider and then Guider in Charge of the 1st Tottenham Ranger Guide Unit attached to the Vale School. When I was Captain, I was determined that this unit would continue doing everything the same as all the able units. Janet, my friend who went on many holidays with me, became my Assistant Guider. It was unlike other clubs for young people with disabilities, which usually entertained their membership, rather than helping them to plan their own activities. I disliked the idea of being seated round a table, facing each other all evening. So for part of the evening I made sure we were all moving around according to our degree of mobility, by taking part in team games. The Guide movement programme allowed us to learn things that would help us to be useful to other people. The girls enjoyed learning first-aid and, more unusually, how to mend a fuse in a plug.

When the unit first started, it relied on voluntary drivers to provide transport to the meetings. Now the council provided transport for those who lived in the borough of Haringey. We had to provide our own escort. Frances answered my letter in the local paper, requesting help in the meetings. She was a teacher and became a valuable helper.

Most girls had cerebral palsy. Danielle had cerebral palsy and spina bifida. When she first joined us at the age of fourteen, she was still at school. She could walk quite well with the aid of crutches. Sadly her disability deteriorated considerably during the years she was with us. Danielle was French and had a lovely family of two sisters and a brother. She was the youngest. I loved visiting her home because I always had a warm welcome. Danielle didn't live very far from me. She had dark, curly hair and was always smiling.

Christine, Danielle's friend, was the only ranger who admitted to being interested in boys. She told us stories about her new boyfriend and I wasn't sure whether or not she was fantasising. We listened with interest during our cup of tea or coffee break during the meeting. 'I've got a new boyfriend, he's called Dave,' Christine said, 'I met him at my club. We're going to the cinema this weekend.'

Noreen had cerebral palsy too. She lived with her aunt in Tottenham and her mother lived in Ireland. It was probable that Noreen's family hoped that she would get better treatment and support in London. She went home to Ireland several times a year and often visited Lourdes. We teased her about all the holidays she had. She had a lovely chuckle and smile. All the Rangers had a marvellous sense of humour.

Maureen, one of the older girls, wanted to be a Ranger forever! It was hard for me to tell her when it was time to leave the Rangers at thirty. Able-bodied Rangers left at twenty. Maureen was able to walk holding on to somebody's arm. She was very enthusiastic to do everything, seeing it as a challenge. She often said, 'Let me have a go.' When it was time for her to leave, I arranged for her to join the Trefoil Guild, in Enfield. I think she settled down with them quite well.

It concerned me that everybody rushed to pick up the girls if they fell over. I hated being swept up from the floor in haste when I fell. I suggested to my helpers that they should let people get up at their own pace after falling. I wanted my helpers to take time to find out the best way of helping the girls get up after a fall. This worked very well.

We had several outings a year. We took part in County Ranger Guides competitions, which involved dressing up and making things. Frances was an invaluable help and had lots of ideas for competitions.

Although I never fulfilled my ambition to be a teacher, at least I was able to introduce some of my own ideas on how best to help young people with disabilities.

While working for HDC I became much more politically aware of disability issues. I'd been on the committee of the North London Spastics' Association for a few years, as their only disabled member.

I became very uncomfortable about the way the committee conducted its business. Its membership

175

was made up of very few people directly associated with cerebral palsy. There was one mother whose son had cerebral palsy. The regional committee of the Spastics Society sent a representative. We also had a social worker from the organisation. The rest of the membership came from varied backgrounds. The treasurer was a local bank manager.

I was particularly uncomfortable about the way the committee discussed grant applications from individual members. There was little attention to confidentiality in the way cases were discussed by a large group of fifteen people. I discussed my concerns with colleagues at work. Many of us felt that the committee should have a greater representation of people with cerebral palsy. In the following months leading up to the AGM several friends offered themselves for election onto the committee. I stood for election as Chairperson. We all got elected onto the committee with me as Chairperson, and Hugh Farrel as Vice Chairperson. It was a complete turn-around of membership status. There was now a large representation of members with cerebral palsy on the committee.

One of the first things I did was to suggest setting up a sub-committee to deal with grant applications. The committee would include Hugh and me, and at least four other committee members, including the treasurer. The few remaining able-bodied members took their revenge. They arranged for the sub-committee to meet at the bank manager's premises in Swiss Cottage at 5.30 p.m., making it impossible for Hugh and me to attend the meeting because we both worked for HDC in Tottenham. However, I was able to take 'Chair's action' and rearrange the venue for future sub-committee meetings to be held at HDC after work. It was a much more sensitive way of dealing with grant applications.

I used to cringe as I listened to the way individual people were discussed by the large committee. 'This poor mother is a single parent, living on income support with her incontinent son John. She's in desperate need of a new washing machine.' This was one committee member's comment after a visit to the applicant's home.

Things would now be done differently. We would continue to help people in a less patronising way and pay much more attention to confidentiality.

The next task for my new committee was to look for a new treasurer as the former one had resigned. He'd existed under the influence of a few patronising committee members whose empire had been overthrown. We wrote to a number of building societies in Haringey inviting an applicant to become treasurer. Two managers offered themselves to stand for election. Stan was duly elected as our new treasurer.

The next step in our revolution was to change the name of our association from North London Spastics' Association to North London Cerebral Palsy Association. Our new name was voted for at our next AGM and was wholeheartedly accepted. We changed our name before the Spastics Society changed their name to Scope. We were involved in discussions to choose a new name for the Spastics Society. I was Chairperson of the local group for about four years. Reluctantly, I had to give up when my parents became ill.

28
A Break from Caring

Rena had her own volunteer called Joan who came into the office once a week. With the introduction of the computer there was less work for her to do. Eventually she became my volunteer. My work was expanding, making it necessary for me to make home visits to people who couldn't get to the office. At first, I made these visits on my own. It was very tiring and time consuming but very worthwhile. But I was beginning to get arthritic pains in my back and was glad of Joan's help accompanying me on these visits.

Margaret Riley, the manager, was a workaholic. She was always in work when the staff arrived in the mornings at 9.30 a.m., and when we left to go home at 5.30 p.m. she was often still working. I admired her dedication to retain a high profile for the HDC. However, it was very hard for a worker with a disability to match the energy and hours she put into her work. Although there were a few applicants with disabilities I was disappointed that a manager with a disability hadn't been appointed. Margaret was partly chosen because she was a carer. I soon realised she was only a carer on her own terms at weekends. I had the impression that she never allowed her care duties to her disabled mother and elderly father to interfere with her work or social life.

Margaret wanted even more elaborate statistics, supplying more information about the kind of people I was advising and the type of advice I was giving. She even demanded a form of contract between me and the person I was helping, with an estimate of how long it would take to complete the work. I very much resented the time spent on all this paperwork as it gave me less time to spend with the client, even though my hours had been extended from 17.5 to 21 hours a week.

Life had much improved at home since I'd had carers looking after Mum and Dad for several hours while I was at work. My sister Margaret also spent one afternoon a week with them. She arranged for her mother-in-law to pick up her children from school. She also did the hospital trips with Mum. She regularly attended the diabetic clinic. It was hard work because she had to keep an eye on Dad, who also came with them to the hospital, as he kept wandering off.

There were times when I had to attend meetings at home with social workers regarding Mum and Dad. It was difficult to get time off for this. Margaret insisted I made the time up. This was difficult because I only worked part-time. Fortunately I had a number of hours left to take off in lieu of the hours when I attended evening meetings.

We had a lovely Chairperson named Moira at this time. She'd just become a grandmother. One day she brought her granddaughter into the office. She was only a few weeks old and very tiny. I was having my lunch-break and, without a word, she placed the baby on my shoulder. I was amazed. How wonderful of her to have left her precious grandchild in my care. It was the first time I'd held a baby on my shoulder. She breathed soft, short little breaths into my ear. It was a wonderful sensation and suddenly all my stress left me.

After that little Paige often came into the office to see me and I always made sure I spent a little time with her. Moira said it was very therapeutic to hold a baby and I agreed. I looked forward so much to seeing this little baby and holding her. It became an oasis in my tense situation. Afterwards whenever I saw a friend with a young baby I automatically held my arms out to take the child. I was disappointed because very few people trusted me to hold a tiny baby. I shall never forget Moira's kindness at this awful time.

The first Christmas we had carers, Mum became poorly with cystitis. She would try to get out of bed during the night to reach the toilet, and fall over. It was becoming very hard for her to get up again. I had to call a doctor out several times. I didn't want to have her admitted into hospital over Christmas. Mum became very dehydrated and she seemed too weak to sit up in bed properly to take her drink. Dad didn't seem to know how to help her. He would have to be my hands. 'Dad, get a dessert spoon and use it to feed Mum with some tea,' I said, crouching on my knees near the radiator just inside the bedroom door wearing my cosy pyjamas. It was a very cold night. I was in a good position to see what was going on. 'That's right Dad, give her some more, perhaps you had better get a small towel from the airing cupboard to catch the drips.' The next day the doctor called again, Mum was desperate to go to the toilet. Dad had popped out. 'Please could you help Mum to the toilet, doctor. She's very weak and needs help to walk. She keeps falling.' The doctor kindly helped her to the toilet and waited for her to finish before assisting her back to bed.

We couldn't visit Margaret and her family for our usual Christmas dinner and tea. I arranged for a carer to stay with Mum and Dad on Christmas Day so that I could join the family. After Christmas, Mum was still poorly. Dad and I were exhausted, so I agreed for Mum to be admitted into hospital for a few days.

While she was there, Dad became very restless and more difficult to look after. We took him to see Mum as often as we could. He missed her very much. It was obvious I wouldn't be able to look after Dad by myself. Fortunately a social worker arranged for him to stay in a local residential home until Mum was discharged from hospital. One evening, as I was settling down to some peace and quiet after a very stressful Christmas period, I heard a knock on my door. Dad had escaped from the home and managed to find his way home again! There was nothing I could do except telephone my sister who came to take him back to the home. There wasn't even a bed made up for him at our home. After Mum fell so ill, everything had to be washed and aired. I felt so sad having to turn my Dad away from his own home.

When Mum was discharged from hospital Margaret brought Dad home on the same day. Mum arrived home first by ambulance. She wanted to know where Dad was. I couldn't tell her the truth. I just said he was with Margaret and on his way home.

It got a little bit too much for me to spend four days at home with Mum and Dad. A carer, named Charm, came to my rescue. I employed her privately on Saturdays for a six-hour period. It made a great difference to my weekend. Charm was such a cheerful person and it was so good to have someone to share the caring. She cooked a roast lunch under my instructions. It was usually steak, one of Mum's favourites. Often, after lunch, Charm took me out in my wheelchair for an hour. Saturdays became enjoyable once again.

I had to supervise Dad increasingly as time went on. I reminded him to have his shower. If left alone, he would put the same clothes back on after he'd worn them the day before. While he was in the shower I went into his bedroom, took the dirty clothes away and put a complete clean set of clothing out for him. He always had money and other things in his trouser pockets. It took time to transfer everything to the clean trousers. There was also a belt to wear with a clean pair of trousers. All this seemed to take an age. I was very nervous while I was doing it, in case he came out of the shower before I'd finished.

As summer approached, I thought Mum and Dad should go on holiday. I knew a place in Cliftonville in Kent that would provide a lovely holiday for them. There was even transport provided from our home. I booked for them to go, and they seemed to look forward to a seaside holiday. Margaret came on the day they were leaving to help them get ready and see them off. I was at work. It was a very hot day. Dad was missing when Margaret arrived. He was out for quite a while. Margaret was very worried and went out looking for him. She found him walking down Muswell Hill, about twenty minutes' walk away, very hot and exhausted. Mum had sent him to the bank for some money to go on holiday. Of course, I'd arranged for them to have enough money for their stay. He needn't have gone all the way to Muswell Hill. He'd obviously forgotten that there was a branch much nearer home. Fortunately, he was home in time to go off on holiday with Mum, and they had a lovely time.

29
Severance

One morning when the foot care lady called to see Mum, she wasn't very happy about Mum's foot. She said that Mum would have to have a home visit from a chiropodist as soon as possible.

At about 7 p.m. that evening, Mum suddenly collapsed. She couldn't pick herself up. I telephoned my GP who seemed to expect my call.

'I'll call an ambulance,' she said, 'You must come to the surgery straight away and collect a letter to take to the hospital.'

Taken aback I asked her, 'But what if the ambulance turns up before I get back?' She replied that the ambulance wouldn't come that quickly.

'Will you please bring the note out to my car to save time?' I said, and was pleased when she agreed to do so.

I couldn't just go away and leave Mum and Dad on their own. I climbed up two flights of stairs to a neighbour and asked if she would stay with Mum and Dad while I went to the surgery.

I managed to get back home before the ambulance arrived but I had to let Mum go on her own to the Whittington Hospital, Highgate. I let Margaret know what had happened.

I didn't get any further information about Mum until the following day. They'd amputated her foot to stop the spread of gangrene. Ten days later, they amputated the same leg up to the knee. When I visited Mum in hospital, she didn't acknowledge that she'd lost her leg.

When she was well enough, they tried to teach her to walk with the use of crutches but she wasn't able to use them. It slowly dawned on us that Mum would never be able to walk or come home again. The hospital staff suggested she needed to be placed in a nursing home.

It affected Dad very badly. He missed her very much. Once again, he had to be placed in residential care. Again he escaped from the care home and turned up at our home. By this time he had been to several residential homes in the borough. Mum had stayed with him in some of them to enable me to have a short break. Some homes refused to re-admit Dad into their care as he'd proved difficult to look after.

Margaret and I took it in turns to take him to visit Mum at least three times a week. When we collected him from the home the staff bombarded us with a torrent of complaints about Dad, speaking as if he were a very naughty child. It was very stressful for Margaret and me. All Dad really wanted was to be with Mum and he

186

didn't know how to reach her. After visiting her he soon forgot his visit and wanted to return to see her again.

All this stress caused severe pain in my neck. My rheumatologist arranged for me to borrow a machine to massage my neck to relieve the tension. As I couldn't put it on myself, a friend and neighbour came at an arranged time each evening to help me to put it on. I had to set a control panel at a speed that felt comfortable. As soon as I had it fixed and was starting to enjoy the relief, there was a knock at the door. Dad had escaped yet again and arrived home. In my panic to turn off the machine and release myself from it, I often turned it too high and got myself into a state.

The police usually brought Dad home. By this time he was in a care home in Potters Bar, roughly 14 miles from home.

'Your Dad cannot possibly escape from Cooper's Croft, it has special locks,' a social worker said. So what was he doing here, I thought.

Apparently he used to stand by the main entrance, wait for somebody to come in or out and then slip out before the door closed again. It wasn't far from the main road to London. He waited and thumbed a lift. Of course, nobody guessed there was anything wrong with him. He could give his address to a willing driver, or the police who offered him a lift. I spent some tense evenings waiting for him to turn up at home. It was heartbreaking to have to tell the sad situation to the police, and explain why I couldn't let him back into his home. After doing this a few times, he was sectioned after being found lying in the road. It was obviously a cry for help. He was admitted to Frien Hospital for the mentally ill, and remained there for about a month.

Margaret and I took it in turns to visit him in the hospital on separate days. We also took him to see Mum who was still in hospital. Margaret and I had no quality time with Mum on our own. Mum was constantly being moved to different wards, while both social services and the NHS were trying to find a suitable nursing home for her. Every time they moved Mum, she deteriorated mentally. The moves upset her.

'Where the hell have you been?' she shouted at Dad on one occasion. 'Out with another woman, I suppose.' Then Dad started swearing at her. It was most embarrassing. We had to end the visits sharply because of the racket they made. Mum and Dad were married for over fifty years. Margaret had given them a lovely Golden Wedding party. The nurses told us that Mum was always calling Dad's name. It was sad to see how much they missed each other, Mum calling him, Dad trying desperately to get to her.

It was very upsetting taking Dad back to the home alone. It was easier when I employed Charm on Saturdays, and she came with me to Potters Bar to collect Dad to take him to see Mum. Her invaluable support helped to relieve much of my stress.

After Dad had been in Frien Barnet Hospital for about a month the registrar told my sister that Dad would have to be returned home as he wasn't really mentally ill and was taking up a much-needed hospital bed.

'After all,' she said, 'your Dad has every right to be in his own home. If your sister doesn't like being at home with him, why doesn't she leave?'

This remark shows how little understanding there was of our family situation. A social worker asked me to visit a list of private nursing homes in the area, and choose one for Dad.

I heard about an excellent home belonging to the NHS situated in St. Ann's Hospital in Tottenham. I rang my doctor, told her about the proposed discharge and asked her about the possibility of placing my Dad in this home.

'He's out of the catchment area,' she replied.

'What are we going to do, doctor? Where can he go?' I asked with concern.

'I don't know, he can't stay in my flat!' she replied.

I was furious. 'Dad doesn't want to stay in his own home,' I said. 'What makes you think that he will stay in your flat?'

I was so upset and angry. It was obvious that everybody thought I was making a fuss over nothing, and didn't want anything to do with caring for my Dad any more. All I wanted was proper care for him in a safe environment, preferably in a home that could also look after Mum.

A week later my sister and I were informed of my father's discharge. It was a Monday, one of the three days that I worked. Margaret went to collect him and brought him home an hour or so before I was expected home from work. We'd arranged to leave him in the charge of Betty, a care attendant who was coming to cook my evening meal. Dad seemed very pleased to be home. Margaret made him a cup of tea and for ten minutes he sat relaxed in an armchair. Then he got up abruptly and made his way towards the front door.

'Where are you going, Dad?' Margaret asked.

'I'm going to see Mum, of course,' he said.

Margaret persuaded him to sit down again and switched on the television for him. After a few minutes he stood up and made for the front door again. Repeatedly, he grew more and more restless. It was time for Margaret to leave. She'd intended to be home by now to give her children their tea. They were being cared for by a friend. Betty refused to stay with Dad on her own. Margaret waited for me to come home and then left. Dad and I had our evening meal. Betty left at her usual time. Dad got up and went outside the flat, saying he was going to see Mum. I couldn't stop him. He came back a few times. He banged the door with his fist impatiently because I couldn't open the door fast enough. It began to get dark as he continued to go in and out of the flat. I put on some lights.

A few minutes later, the police arrived at the door.

'We have had a report of a burglary. Is everything alright?' A policeman asked.

I was puzzled. 'Yes,' I replied. 'I live here. Everything's fine.'

Apparently, when Dad had seen lights on in the flat, he'd gone to the hospital across the road and told somebody there were burglars in his flat. Dad continued to go in and out and I grew more and more frustrated.

Twice a neighbour brought him home again, saying, 'Could you try and keep your father indoors? He's making himself a nuisance coming to my flat and mistaking it for his.'

I decided to double-lock the front door to keep Dad in and rang my GP.

'Give your Dad his medication and a warm, milky drink,' she advised. 'Put the lights out. Then he'll go to bed thinking its bedtime.'

Little did she know that I had difficulty making myself a hot drink, let alone making one for Dad. Instead, I supervised him making himself a cup of tea and he took his medication.

I began to feel more relaxed, thinking the medication would help him to fall asleep easily. I'd hidden the front door keys in case he tried to go outside again.

30
Some Drastic Action

I heard Dad dialling 999 for the fire brigade. He told them he couldn't unlock his front door. I was horrified. All I could do was wait for them to arrive and explain to them what had happened. When they arrived, I tried to persuade them to phone my doctor to see if I could get him re-admitted into hospital. They took down the details but took no action. It was time for bed so I hid every key in the flat before retiring to bed, hoping Dad would do the same.

I had very little sleep that night. All night long, Dad tried to open the front door with scissors, knives and screwdrivers. He was so determined. He kept coming into my bedroom asking me for the front door keys. He became quite threatening at times and I thought he might hit me. I felt safer lying down in my bed. I heard him go into the kitchen several times to make himself some tea. I was worried in case he might cause a fire or leave the gas on. When I smelt gas during the night, I ventured into the kitchen and found a gas tap on. Dad finally fell asleep at 5 a.m.

Margaret called the next morning and found me exhausted and very distressed. I phoned the social worker to tell her of the terrible happenings in the night.

'Have you found a suitable home for your father?' she asked. 'Arrange for him to be admitted. Social Services will cover the cost.'

I'd found a private home. Margaret and her husband took Dad along to it later that day. The manager promised that they would take good care of Dad and wouldn't let him escape.

Five days later the manager called me to tell me what a terrible time they were having trying to prevent him from escaping. He thought the best way to help Dad and the family was just to let him escape from the home. They would give him his belongings packed in his suitcase. Showing some concern, he persuaded me that by taking this drastic course of action the police would pick Dad up and take him back to Frien Hospital. I was at work when I received a phone call from the police.

'We have your Dad here, Madam. We have instructions to take him to your home. Will you please meet us there with your keys to let him in?'

I had already told Margaret that if I were forced to look after Dad again I would refuse. I intended to leave home, leaving him to his own devices. I felt I had to prove to the authorities that Dad couldn't look after himself. There was no way I could stay home from work to be with him all the day and night. Margaret

194

agreed with my proposed course of action and invited me to come and stay with her.

I went home as the police requested and let Dad in. A policeman and woman were waiting for me with Dad. I told them I would not be able to stay with him. I asked them to stay with us while I packed my things to leave.

Dad followed me around the flat as I packed. saying, 'Don't go, Joan, don't leave me.'

I gave him a spare key. He followed me to my car and knocked on the window with his fist. It was horrible. I was nearly in tears as I resisted his pleas. The policeman and woman looked visibly upset too.

The next day I informed social services and the GP that I'd left Dad at home and was staying with my sister. Social Services arranged for him to have meals-on-wheels delivered and for a home help to call and give him his medication. He was rarely at home when they came. A neighbour telephoned Margaret to complain about the havoc Dad was causing. Others took him in and gave him tea. Another neighbour went to stay at home with him and tried to settle him down to sleep. He spent one night in a care home.

Dad was convinced Mum was in the small hospital opposite. He weaved in between heavy traffic to cross the road. It was very dangerous. Four days later Margaret and I went home. Dad wasn't in but he arrived a few minutes later. Margaret found out that Dad's keys were being held in the hospital opposite.

On arrival at the hospital Margaret was in time to join a meeting called by the manager to discuss Dad's predicament. We hadn't known about this meeting. Dad's GP and the geriatrician from Frien Hospital were there. Nobody offered a solution. There were long silences.

Then the geriatrician piped up. 'If it was my father I'd take him anywhere.' Margaret replied sternly, 'Tell me where I can take Dad and I'll take him there.' Finally, the geriatrician agreed to admit Dad back into his hospital until a better solution was found.

The following week Margaret and I were called to attend a meeting at Frien Hospital to discuss our parents' future care. I'd given much thought to what I wanted to say at this meeting. Seated around a large table were representatives from the NHS who were caring for both Mum and Dad, some Social Services staff and Dad's geriatrician who chaired the meeting.

Before anyone spoke I insisted on having my say.

> 'I hope what I have to say will set the agenda for this meeting. For fifty-three years I've lived in a body that has caused total chaos in my world through my disability. My Dad, for his part, has always tried to make life as easy for me as possible and made all kinds of gadgets to assist my independence. When Dad developed an illness that stopped him making sense of his world, I did my best to help him overcome his difficulties, but today we have both reached a point where we can no longer help

each other. The consequences of placing us both under the same roof is to double our respective disabilities.' I paused and then concluded by saying, 'I hope that there is enough humanity and expertise among you all to find a solution to Mum and Dad's future care.'

There was silence as I spoke, followed by a short discussion on what kind of care was required. Mum needed special nursing care and Dad needed constant supervision. It was agreed at the meeting that every effort should be made to find a suitable home that would make this provision for both parents. Lack of money was a considerable problem that hindered the provision of proper care.

A few weeks later Margaret and I were called to Mum's bedside. She was already in a coma and never came out of it. Margaret fetched Dad and we stayed with her for as long as we could. It was a very cold and wet November evening. Mum died a few hours after we left her.

The whole ward was about to be moved to a new nursing home attached to the little hospital opposite. Dad wasn't going to be put there. I was glad that Mum didn't have to face another move because I knew how badly it would have affected her.

Dad was eventually transferred to the home attached to St. Ann's Hospital in Tottenham, the one I'd asked my GP about. He lived for two and a half years. It was a lovely home. The staff were wonderfully kind. Margaret and I visited him two or three times a week on different days. Margaret often took him home for a couple of hours on a Sunday afternoon.

On my visits I took him a bag of sweets from the Pick-'n-Mix counter in Woolworths. They were wrapped up and we each took one out of the bag.

Dad looked at me. 'I'll take the paper off for you,' he said.

I handed my sweet to him. It was touching to see that he hadn't forgotten I needed help. As time went on he found it harder to unwrap the sweet and handed it back to me with his own. I had to unwrap both sweets. I'd noticed members of staff watching him helping me. I was pleased that they'd seen this side of his nature. He became unstable on his feet. When I got up to walk, he instinctively linked his arm though mine to help me. One day, we both fell over!

Dad often asked me on my visits, 'Did you come by car? Where is it parked? Is it far away?'

I knew what he was thinking. When it was time to leave, he would try to come with me but the ward was locked. The staff watched him as I left to make sure he didn't follow me. He couldn't believe what had happened to him.

He often asked, 'Is this a dream?' If so, it was a horrible dream.

One day Margaret and I were called to his bedside. He died peacefully. We were so thankful for the wonderful care he received in the end. It was a great pity that it was such a battle to get it. I wouldn't wish this situation on anyone.

31
Vancouver and Susy from Hackney

Jill, one of my friends in Guides and Rangers, emigrated to Canada soon after she got married. She had always kept in touch with me, writing to me at least twice a year. When she came home to England she nearly always called on me. It was my dream that one day I would visit her for a holiday.

I fulfilled this dream the year after Mum died. I was pretty confident that Frances, my assistant from Brownies, would come with me and was delighted when she agreed. I wrote to Jill and her husband Bob, about our proposed three week visit and asked if they knew of good accommodation where we could stay. Jill wrote back insisting we stay with her and Bob. We took nearly a year to plan our trip.

Apparently May was the best month to visit, being the beginning of summer. We were very fortunate in having beautiful weather for the whole three weeks. Vancouver seemed to have everything in one place – snow capped mountains and sandy beaches.

It was a nine hour flight from Gatwick so I was very stiff for the first few days, even though I did try to walk a little in the plane. Bob was our chauffeur/guide throughout the holiday as he had taken early retirement but Jill was at work all day teaching in a local school.

One of the first things that struck me about Vancouver was the number of people with disabilities on the streets and waiting at the bus stops. Many of them travelled around on electric scooters. Before coming to Canada, I had seen very few people using electric scooters in London. Here in Canada the access for people with disabilities was amazing. All public transport had wheelchair access, even the monorail. It was great to be able to get into a lift at pavement level and be transported up to the monorail. Canada had already passed the Disability Discrimination Act, putting into place a law that ensured all public buildings and transport are wheelchair accessible. Ten years later we passed a similar Act in Britain in November 2004.

Frances and I wanted to have a little adventure on our own on the second weekend. We decided to go to Seattle for the weekend. Crossing over to the USA required a special visa so Bob escorted us to the US border and to the local travel agent to book accommodation and transport. We went to Seattle by coach. It was very exciting planning it all. I was amazed how easy it was to book wheelchair accessible rooms in the hotel. They were actually a little cheaper than the other rooms! We had a wonderful weekend sight-seeing on a special tram. We were able to get on and off whenever we wished to see different places. One area of Seattle had quite a few small art galleries and we visited most of them.

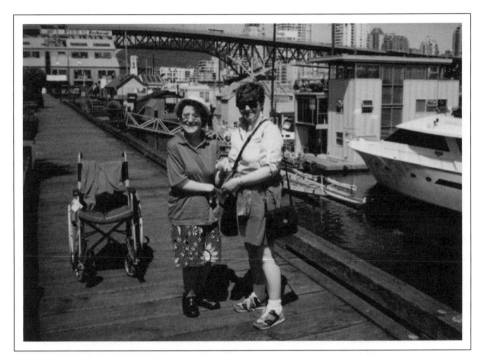

Frances and myself at Granville Island in 1994.

Jill and Bob also organised a weekend trip for Frances and me to Vancouver Island. We went by boat, which took about two hours. We stayed two nights in Victoria, the capital of the island. Jill and Bob joined us on the Sunday and took us to the other side of the island on the pacific coast. The scenery was breathtaking on this part of the island. The lakes were so clear containing the reflections of the snow-capped mountains. This part of the island also had the tallest pine trees I've ever seen. There were also large areas left very barren after the destruction of forest fires. It was quite frightening to imagine the devastation these fires caused on such a vast scale.

In the mornings, whilst sitting on the veranda waiting for Bob to return from shopping, I made friends with their dark ginger cat who often came on my lap. I hadn't had much to do with cats before but I took a great fancy to this cat. Frances often said to me, "I think we'll have an extra piece of luggage going home!" implying that I was thinking of smuggling this dear little cat back home with me to England.

This was indeed an unforgettable holiday. Jill and Bob were the perfect hosts. Frances too was a wonderful companion. Some eleven years after we are still talking about this holiday whenever we meet.

Two things happened as a result of my trip to Vancouver.

First, I decided I must definitely get myself an electric scooter to enable me to go out and about locally. I acquired a scooter within a year. It certainly did change my life. I could take the scooter to places I couldn't get to by car, into the park on sunny days and into the larger shops, providing there was good access. I could browse for much longer without getting tired from standing too long. I had to keep my scooter in my garage, which was quite a difficult walk as I got older and became arthritic. I had to wait two years for the council to build me a ramp enabling me to put my scooter into a shed a few yards from my flat.

Second, I acquired Susy, a black and white kitten of eleven weeks old.

My sister, Margaret, had a friend who needed to house a kitten. Susy was one of a litter of five kittens, all black and white. She had the most white in her and was the only female. I didn't know much about cats but I thought she would be easier to look after, as I had the impression that tomcats are always rather large.

Susy arrived on a Friday evening, in a little cardboard box, carefully sealed. I had everything ready for her. I bought a small litter tray. A cardboard box with some old jumpers in it made a very cosy bed under the kitchen table.

Susy was placed on my lap. Margaret's friend told me it was the first time she had stayed on somebody's lap. I had a photo taken with her. We had already bonded. Left alone with her, the weight of taking care of this little thing was quite a responsibility. "What if I hurt her when I pick her up? I can't hold her the way it tells you to in the cat care book," I said to Margaret. "Oh you'll find a way of doing it," Margaret said reassuringly.

I gave Susy some special milk for kittens. It was a powder that was mixed with water. Italia used to make up a bottle for me and leave it in the fridge. One of the first times she had it I poured the milk into a saucer but my arm made an involuntary spasm and the milk went all over Susy instead! She spent the next 15 minutes or so washing herself. "Well Susy, that's what it's like being looked after by somebody with cerebral palsy. It's something you'll have to get used to I'm afraid."

I had started having carers in on the mornings that I worked because it was becoming more difficult to make my own breakfast and getting out by a certain time. I was concerned that my carer would open the kitchen balcony door, forgetting about Susy, and she would escape.

I used to get very worried if she was out too long. If she hadn't turned up home again after two or three hours I was nearly in tears. It worried me that I couldn't walk around outside and pick her up if I saw her and take her home again. Once or twice I went round on my scooter looking for her and calling her name, only to come home and find her waiting for me on the kitchen windowsill. I realised it was a waste of time to go and look for her. You just couldn't see a black and white cat in the bushes or trees. I don't know how she managed to camouflage herself so well.

It was amazing how Susy has adapted to my disability. She always comes to my left side to be stroked because I always used my left hand. She never rubs against my legs when I am standing or walking but always waits until I am sitting down. She is a great companion. I wouldn't be without her. When I haven't seen her for a while, and call her, she will usually come and see me just to reassure me that she isn't far away.

Epilogue

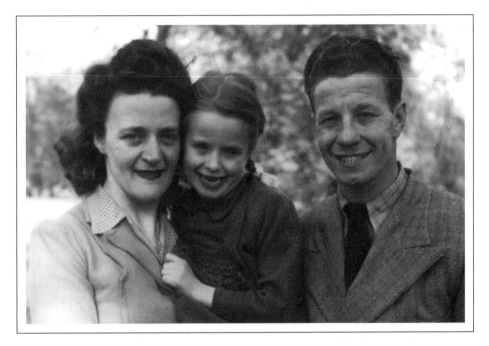

Out and about with Mum and Dad when he came on leave, 1946.

The baby whose parents were told she might grow up not recognising her parents didn't do so badly after all. Although I wasn't allowed to fulfil my ambition to become a teacher, I was privileged with countless opportunities to work with children.

My life-story is like a tapestry where everything fits together for a purpose. Each experience taught me something and prepared me for something bigger. Having to overcome difficult situations made me a stronger person. I never felt alone in my struggles as I always sensed God's presence guiding me. He kept His promise by not giving me anything too difficult to bear, without the strength and support to overcome it.

I have met some wonderful, caring people during my life. They were always the right people who met my special needs in difficult times. I believe that God doesn't just use Christians to do His work. All kinds of people are used to fulfil His purpose.

I regard my parents as being remarkable in recognising my potential even as a baby. My mother disregarded the doctor's prognosis of severe brain damage. She searched out the best treatment for me and insisted that I should be educated. Her determination to allow me the freedom to live life to the full was infectious, encouraging others to assist me in the same way.

I value those friends with physical disabilities who taught me so much. Sylvia, my childhood friend married Tom who had a disability. They have a daughter and are extremely proud of their grandson, Bradley. Life hasn't been easy for them. Sylvia is fighting hard to remain independent, despite health problems related to age. The couple lived close to Sylvia's parents, and cared for them as they aged. Tom runs a social club in Enfield, and they both do charity work.

Janet moved to Cambridge with her parents about fifteen years ago. We stopped going on holidays together because of Janet's failing health. She comes to stay with me for weekends several times a year. She borrows my scooter so she can browse around the shops in Crouch End. I miss our holidays together but was fortunate to find the Winged Fellowship Trust's group holiday schemes that helped me to travel mostly abroad.

In 1991, the year Mum died, my sister Margaret gained a BSc Honours degree in New Technology as a mature student, and moved house. Sadly our parents were too ill to appreciate Margaret's achievements. Earlier on they would have been so proud of her. She went on to teach Business Studies at Hackney Community College.

Auntie Madge and Uncle Karol retired and moved to Holyhead. Uncle Karol lived to be ninety. Auntie became ill with dementia a few years after my father died. Once again Margaret and I were involved in a serious family illness. For a year Margaret had to travel to Wales every month, taking full responsibility for our aunt's affairs until she died. It was a horrible time for her.

It's ironic that, as a young girl, I was considered too disabled to do the things I longed to do. Attitudes changed when my parents needed my care, and my severe disability was disregarded. Yet, being a carer enabled me to empathise with other carers in my work as an Advice Officer, and they and others appreciated this. In 1999 I was made redundant nine months before I would have retired. The Management Committee, persuaded that financial cuts were necessary, disbanded the advice service. It wasn't a coincidence that the manager, Steve, who'd succeeded Margaret Riley, had asked me three weeks prior to this to exchange offices with him. Although I sympathised with his poor working conditions, I'd refused because his office was too small to hold interviews with people in wheelchairs, their carers and often an interpreter. The office had no natural daylight and overlooked a busy railway track with noisy trains. The thin partitioned walls offered little privacy for dealing with distressed people and confidential matters.

I felt Steve had little regard for my advice work. He wasn't interested in my statistics. Given my redundancy notice, I was told of plans to place specialist advisers on disability at advice bureaux in the borough, but it never happened. At the time, I had thirty complex cases on my list and had to call people in to return their files.

'We don't want to queue up for hours at an advice bureau,' they said. 'Please can we visit you at home?' Sadly, this wasn't possible.

In the year I left work, Peter, my brother-in-law, found out that he had lung cancer. It was devastating news. He'd never smoked. The chemicals he'd used when he first worked as a graphic artist were a likely cause. He bravely fought his illness for three cruel years. Although hardly mentioned in my story, he was like a brother to me. He was so kind and gentle, and always supported all my adventures. He often had me in fits of laughter and I miss him very much.

To be born with impairment or to be struck down by illness is a tragedy. People deal with it in different ways. There are many examples of how people turn things around and make good of their plight. I've been asked many times how having a disability affects me. Would I like to be normal? It would feel a little strange. I mostly accept my disability as a challenge. It's the hostile environment and attitudes of others that disables me.

Two things happened that jolted me into realising, unconsciously, that I didn't want to be disabled. A few years ago, I attended a friend's funeral. Peter had been very disabled. He'd died suddenly, and it was very sad. During the funeral service, a thought came to me: 'Peter isn't disabled anymore, he has a new body and a new life!' I felt excited and happy for him. It surprised me that I was harbouring such a deep-rooted resentment of disability.

Recently, I've been profoundly moved by a very clear image of a baby in a womb. The baby moves around, using her limbs normally. I was looking at myself as a normal baby before I was born. It was a very emotional experience.

Now I have a second disability: osteoarthritis. It's given me a whole new experience of inactivity because of severe pain in my arms, shoulders and neck. I have always been grateful cerebral palsy wasn't painful, apart from the occasional muscle sprain. I can handle cerebral palsy much better than arthritis. In the past, there was always a way of overcoming physical difficulties. I taught myself easier and different ways of doing things. But it doesn't work like that with arthritis. Pain is now the master of my life. Either I give into it, and cut down on my activities, or I defy it and insist on doing my normal activities or at least some of them. This results in increased pain and tiredness. Hopefully, shoulder replacement surgery will be able to reduce the severe pain.

I shall never be able to do some of the activities I learnt to do with so much pleasure in the past. However, it doesn't matter as I don't have to prove myself anymore. I enjoy thinking back on my achievements, and say from the bottom of my heart:

'Praise to God for the abundant life He has given me.'